中英双语版

THE CHARM OF TRADITIONAL CHINESE MEDICINE II

神奇的
中医药

（二）

赵继荣　米登海／主编

王世杰　赵玉华　周丽琴／译

Chief Editors: Zhao Jirong　Mi Denghai

Translators: Wangshijie　Zhao Yuhua　Zhou Liqin

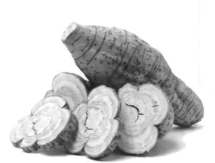

甘肃科学技术出版社

Gansu Science and Technology Press

甘肃·兰州
Lanzhou, Gansu

U0321407

图书在版编目（CIP）数据

　　神奇的中医药：中英双语版．二 / 赵继荣，米登海
主编；王世杰，赵玉华，周丽琴译． -- 兰州：甘肃科
学技术出版社，2024．9． -- ISBN 978-7-5424-3215-5

　　Ⅰ．R2

中国国家版本馆CIP数据核字第20245B1T96号

神奇的中医药（二）（中英双语版）

SHENQI DE ZHONGYIYAO (ER) (ZHONG-YING SHUANGYU BAN)

赵继荣　米登海　主编

王世杰　赵玉华　周丽琴　译

项目策划	朱黎明　杨丽丽	
翻译策划	刘　唱　张艳萍　舒　畅	
译文主审	郭亚银　武永胜	
责任编辑	史文娟	
封面设计	石　璞	

出　版　甘肃科学技术出版社
社　址　兰州市城关区曹家巷1号　730030
电　话　0931-2131575（编辑部）　0931-8773237（发行部）

发　行　甘肃科学技术出版社　　印　刷　甘肃兴业印务有限公司
开　本　787毫米×1092毫米 1/16　印　张　14　插　页　1　字　数　196千
版　次　2024年9月第1版
印　次　2024年9月第1次印刷
印　数　1~2300
书　号　ISBN 978-7-5424-3215-5　　　　定　价　98.00元

出 版 说 明

　　中医药学包含着中华民族几千年的健康养生理念及其实践经验,是中华文明的一个瑰宝,凝聚着中国人民和中华民族的博大智慧。学习中医药文化,可以补充医学知识,培养健康养生理念,启发科学探索,亦可促进国际文化交流。因此,我们策划并出版中医药文化科普图书《神奇的中医药(中英双语版)》系列,以便高校、科研院所的国际交流生、在华生活的外籍人员乃至大众了解中医药文化的渊源和本真。

　　本丛书专为普及中医药文化而作,以提纲挈领的方式,向读者介绍中医药文化的精髓。第一、二册循序渐进,各有侧重。第一册讲述:中医药学的起源与发展、中医药学故事、古今中医药学教育、中医药学对世界的贡献,旨在帮助读者了解中医药学的发展脉络;第二册则涵盖:走近中医药、中医药学蕴藏的智慧、中药与方剂、甘肃中医药故事及生活中的中医保健;旨在帮助读者了解中医药学的理论体系、追溯中医药文化的根源。每本书通过 25 个经典、有趣的故事,将中医药文化娓娓道来。本丛书内容精炼,图文并茂,兼具科学性、通俗性和趣味性。

　　甘肃是中医药文化重要的发祥地之一,在中医药学教育方面也有着深厚的国际交流积淀。作为资深的中医药学者、践行者兼教授,本书作者以系统的思维、清晰的逻辑,深入浅出地向读者介绍中医药及其文化的精髓。在编写和出版过程中,我们进行了深层次的研究和探索,广泛征求意见,反复修改,精益求精,但可能依旧存在疏漏与不足之处,恳请各位老师、同学指正。希冀这套书不断优化,成为中医药文化的优秀双语科普读物,为人们了解中医药文化提供便捷。

PUBLICATION NOTES

Traditional Chinese Medicine (TCM) encompasses the health-preserving philosophy and practical experience of the Chinese nation spanning thousands of years. It is a treasure of Chinese civilization and embodies the accumulated and profound wisdom of the Chinese nation. Studying TCM culture can broaden medical knowledge, foster wellness concepts, inspire scientific exploration, and facilitate cultural exchanges between nations. Therefore, we have planned and published *The Charm of Traditional Chinese Medicine* (*Chinese-English Edition*), a series of popular science books on TCM culture, which is intended to introduce the origin and essence of TCM to international exchange students in Chinese universities and research institutes, foreigners living in China, and the public at large.

This two-book series is specifically designed to popularize TCM culture, presenting the readers with the quintessence of TCM culture in a concise and comprehensive manner. With each book having its own focus, the chapters are gradually and progressively arranged. The first covers the origin and development of TCM, stories or legends about TCM, ancient and modern TCM education, and the contributions of TCM to the world, aiming to make the readers fully informed about the evolutions of TCM. The second contains an introduction to TCM, great wisdom embedded in TCM, numerous medicines and formulas, stories about particular physicians or medicines in Gansu, and TCM healthcare in daily life, aiming to help the readers understand the theoretical system of TCM and the context of TCM culture. Moreover, each book is adequately illustrated with colour pictures and skillfully interspersed with 25 classic and amusing stories or anecdotes about TCM culture. All this makes the books concise and informative as well as readable and absorbing.

Gansu, one of the important birthplaces of TCM culture, boasts considerable experience of international exchange in TCM education. As seasoned scholars, practitioners and professors of TCM, the authors have employed a systematic and logic approach to make a general and popular introduction of the essence of TCM and its culture to the readers. Throughout the compilation and publication of the books, we editors and translators have conducted thorough research and exploration, canvassed diverse opinions, and made repeated revisions, and strived for perfection. However, there may still be omissions, deficiencies or errors, and we kindly ask our readers to point them out. We hope that this series will be improved and finally become an excellent bilingual popular science publication on TCM culture, providing convenience for people interested in TCM culture.

目　录

Contents

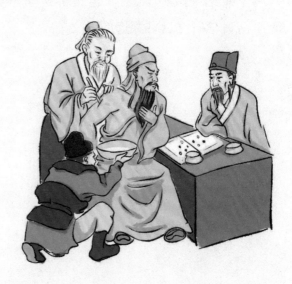

第一单元　走近中医药

中华民族是世界上历史最悠久的民族之一，中医药学是全国各族人民在几千年的生活、生产实践以及与疾病作斗争的过程中逐渐形成并不断发展、丰富的医学科学。毛泽东主席曾经说过："中国医药学是一个伟大的宝库，应当努力发掘，加以提高。"习近平总书记指出："中医药学凝聚着深邃的哲学智慧和中华民族几千年的健康养生理念及其实践经验，是中华文明的一个瑰宝，也是打开中华文明宝库的钥匙。深入研究和科学总结中医药学，对丰富世界医学事业、推进生命科学研究具有深远的意义。"

Unit I Understanding Traditional Chinese Medicine

The Chinese nation is one of the oldest in the world, and Traditional Chinese Medicine (TCM) is a medical science that has been gradually formed, continuously developed and enriched by the people of all nationalities in China in the course of thousands of years of their life, production, and struggle against diseases. Chairman Mao Zedong once said, "Traditional Chinese Medicine is a vast treasure-house of knowledge, deserving to be diligently exploited and refined." President Xi Jinping pointed out: " Traditional Chinese Medicine embodies profound wisdoms and health-preserving concepts as well as practical experience accumulated over thousands of years by the Chinese nation. It is an essential part of Chinese civilization and also a key to gaining access to the treasure house of Chinese civilization. The thorough research and scientific refinement of Traditional Chinese Medicine has tremendous significance for enriching modern medicine and advancing life science research."

　　这一单元主要带领大家穿越时空隧道,一起感悟中医药的博大精深,探寻中医药发展的源头,聆听古代医家的成才故事,领略中医药宝库中的精华,了解现代中医的传承创新,紧跟中医走向世界的步伐,感受中医药学古老而蓬勃的生机与活力。

This unit is designed to lead everyone through the tunnel of time and space to an understanding of the extensive and profound TCM, explore the sources and development of TCM, know about the inspirational stories of ancient physicians, appreciate the essence of TCM and thus comprehend the inheritance and innovation of modern TCM. Let's focus on the spread of TCM to the world, and feel the ancient and booming vitality of TCM.

第一章　源远流长的中医药学

中医药学是在广袤而深厚的中华民族传统文化土壤中孕育而成的,是中华文明的瑰宝。数千年来伴随着中华民族从远古时代走向现代社会,为各族人民的繁衍生息和生命健康保驾护航。

170万年前,中华民族的祖先就已经生息、劳动、繁衍在这片土地上。人们在同自然灾害、猛兽、疾病作斗争的漫长过程中,逐步认识自然,获得知识,渐渐地发现运用身边的一些动植物可以解除病痛。《史记》《淮南子》《搜神记》等众多古书中都记载着"神农尝百草"的动人传说,详细描绘了华夏始祖神农是如何为百姓寻找防治疾病的药物和方法。随着原始社会畜牧业和农业的不断发展,到了夏商时期,人们已经学会通过酿酒和熬制汤药来提高中草药的用药疗效。

Chapter 1 Traditional Chinese Medicine with a Long History

Traditional Chinese Medicine (TCM) nurtured in the extensive and profound Chinese cultural traditions, is a treasure of Chinese civilization. It has accompanied the Chinese nation from ancient times to the modern era, safeguarding the reproduction and health of the people of all nationalities.

About 1.7 million years ago, the ancestors of the Chinese nation began to live, work and multiply on their primitive land. In the long process of fighting against natural disasters, beasts and diseases, people gradually learned about nature, acquired knowledge, and ultimately found that the use of some animal parts and plants around them could help them relieve pain. Many ancient books, such as the *Shi Ji* (*Records of the Grand Historian*), *Huainanzi* (*Great Words from Huainan*), and *Sou Shen Ji* (*Stories of Immortals*), record the moving legend of "Shennong tasting hundreds of herbs", describing in detail how Shennong, a great ancestor of the Chinese people, discovered medicines from herbs and methods to prevent and treat diseases. As primitive society's animal husbandry and agriculture continued to develop, by the time of the Xia and Shang dynasties, people had already begun to explore ways to enhance the efficacy of herbal medicines through the brewing of alcoholic liquids and the making of medicinal decoctions.

春秋战国时期,中医理论已经基本形成,出现了解剖和医学分科,名医扁鹊在总结前人医疗经验的基础上,结合自己的临床实践,创造性地提出了"望、闻、问、切"四诊合参的方法,正式奠定了中医临床诊断和治疗的基础,当时的治疗方法有砭石、针刺、汤药、艾灸、导引等。

During the Spring and Autumn and the Warring States periods, the theories on TCM had been basically formed, and a division of anatomy and medicine appeared. Bianque, a famous doctor, creatively put forward the methods of diagnosis (observing, listening and smelling, inquiring and pulse-taking) by summing up the medical experience of predecessors and combining them with his own clinical practice, which formally laid the foundation for the clinical diagnosis and treatment in TCM. Treatments include treating with healing stone, acupuncture, decoction, moxibustion, daoyin (a regimen in ancient times which combines breathing exercises and body movement), etc.

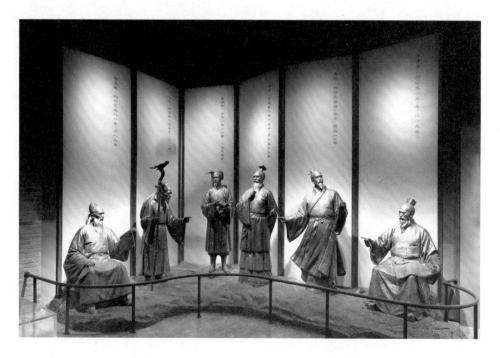

　　战国至秦汉年间,诞生了《黄帝内经》,它是中国传统医学四大经典著作之一,也是中国医学宝库中成书最早的医学典籍之一,标志着中医学理论体系的初步形成。东汉时期出现了著名医学家张仲景,他所著《伤寒杂病论》(后世流传为《伤寒论》和《金匮要略》),将中医的理、法、方、药有机结合,是中国第一部从理论到实践、确立辨证论治法则的临床专著。华佗则以精通外科手术和麻醉名闻天下,还创立了健身体操"五禽戏"。唐代孙思邈总结前人的理论经验,收集了5000多个药方,编著《千金要方》和《千金翼方》,被后人尊为"药王"。

　　金元时期,中医学百家争鸣,出现了"金元四大家"。

　　明清之际,出现了温病学派,对传染性疾病进行了深入研究,明朝后期成书的《本草纲目》被称为"古代中国百科全书"。

Between the Warring States period and the Qin and Han dynasties, the *Huangdi Neijing* (*Huangdi's Classic of Medicine*) was born, which is one of the classics of TCM and the earliest medical books, marking the initial formation of the theoretical system of TCM. In the Eastern Han dynasty, Zhang Zhongjing, a famous physician, wrote the *Shanghan Zabing Lun* (*Treatise on Exogenous Febrile and Miscellaneous Diseases*), later known as the *Shanghan Lun* (*Treatise on Exogenous Febrile Diseases*) and *Jingui Yaolue* (*Essential Prescriptions of the Golden Chamber*). This classic, combining theories, methods and prescriptions, has been honored as the first clinical monograph in China to establish the principle of syndrome differentiation and treatment both theoretically and practically. Hua Tuo, famous for his proficiency in surgery and anesthesia, created the wuqinxi (a set of physical exercises imitating the movements of the five animals). In the Tang dynasty, Sun Simiao, by summarizing the theoretical experience of his predecessors, collected more than 5000 prescriptions and wrote the *Qianjin Yao Fang* (*Invaluable Prescriptions*) and *Qianjin Yi Fang* (*A Supplement to Invaluable Prescriptions*), thus having been hailed as China's king of medicine by later generations.

During the Jin and Yuan dynasties, TCM flourished and different schools sprang up and argued with each other, which gave a rise to the advent of the so called four great medical schools in the Jin and Yuan dynasties.

In the Ming and Qing dynasties, the school of epidemic febrile diseases emerged and it conducted intensive research on infectious diseases. The *Bencao Gangmu* (*A Compendium of Materia Medica*), written by Li Shizhen in the late Ming dynasty, has been called an encyclopedia of ancient China.

中华人民共和国成立以来，党和国家高度重视中医药，并大力支持中医药发展。毛泽东主席曾指出："中国医药学是一个伟大的宝库，应当努力发掘，加以提高。"近年来，党和国家对中医药事业的发展规划步入新的历史时期。习近平总书记指出："中医药学凝聚着深邃的哲学智慧和中华民族几千年的健康养生理念及其实践经验，是中国古代科学的瑰宝，也是打开中华文明宝库的钥匙。"当前，中医药与西医药优势互补，相互促进，共同维护和增进民众健康，已经成为中国特色医药卫生与健康事业的重要特征和显著优势。

2016年《中华人民共和国中医药法》的颁布与实施，标志着第一次从国家法律层面明确了中医药的重要地位、发展方针和扶持措施，这是中医药发展史上具有里程碑意义的大事。党中央、国务院印发了第一个关于中医药工作的专门文件——《关于促进中医药传承创新发展的意见》。国务院召开第一次全国中医药大会，出台一系列促进中医药传承创新发展的重大举措，以前所未有的力度推进中医药改革发展。

Since the founding of the People's Republic of China(PRC), leaders of the Communist Party of China (CPC) and the state have attached great importance to TCM and greatly supported its development. Chairman Mao Zedong once said, "Chinese medicine is a great treasure house well worth being explored and improved." In recent years, the development plan of the CPC and the state for the cause of TCM has entered a new historical period. President Xi Jinping pointed out that TCM embodies profound philosophical wisdom, thousands of years of health preservation concepts and practical experience of the Chinese nation and thus it is a treasure of ancient Chinese science as well as a key to understanding the Chinese civilization. At present, TCM and Western medicine complement and promote each other, and jointly safeguard and improve people's health, which has become an important feature and significant advantage of medical and health undertakings with Chinese characteristics.

In 2016, the *Law of the People's Republic of China on Traditional Chinese Medicine* was promulgated, marking the important position, development policy and support for TCM at the national legal level for the first time and being viewed as a milestone in the history of the development of TCM. The Central Committee of the CPC and the State Council issued the first document on the work of TCM, that is, the *Opinions on Facilitating the Inheritance, Innovation and Development of Traditional Chinese Medicine*. In addition, the State Council held the first national meeting of TCM and introduced a series of new policies to boost the inheritance, innovation and development of TCM, aiming at promoting the reform and improvement of TCM with an unprecedented effort.

在新型冠状病毒感染疫情在全世界流行期间,以《伤寒杂病论》中的经方为基础化裁而成的清肺排毒汤,成为防治新冠病毒感染的重要手段之一,在疫情防控救治的全过程发挥了重要作用。中医药战"疫"经验走出了国门,得到国际社会越来越多的关注和认可,"发挥中医药优势、坚持中西医结合"成为中国方案、中国经验的最显著特征之一。面向未来,中医药学将继续勇攀医学高峰,不断推进自身的现代化和国际化。

Since the global spread of the COVID-19 pandemic, the *Qingfei Paidu Decoction* (a decoction for clearing the lungs and eliminating toxin), which is based on the classical formulas from the *Shanghan Zabing Lun* (*Treatise on Exogenous Febrile and Miscellaneous Diseases*) and adapted for modern use, has become one of the important methods for preventing and treating COVID-19 infections. It has played a significant role throughout the entire process of epidemic prevention, control, and treatment. The experience of TCM in fighting against the epidemic has also spread abroad and received more and more attention and recognition from the international community. "Exploiting the advantage of TCM and adhering to the integration of TCM and Western medicine" has become one of the core features of China's anti-epidemic program and experience. Facing the future, TCM will continue to bravely scale new heights in medicine, constantly promote its modernization and internationalization.

第二章 中医药名家

神医华佗

华佗(约145—208),沛国谯(今安徽亳州)人。东汉末年医学家,精内、儿、针灸各科,外科尤为擅长。他发明的"麻沸散"是世界医学史上最早的麻醉剂,为外科医学的开拓和发展开创了新的研究领域。他的发明比牙科医生摩尔顿发明乙醚麻醉获得成功(1846年)要早1600多年。

Chapter 2 Famous Physicians of Traditional Chinese Medicine

Hua Tuo, a Miracle Doctor

Hua Tuo (circa 145-208 AD), was born in Jiao county, Pei-guo (now Bozhou, Anhui province). As a physician at the end of the Eastern Han dynasty, he specialized in internal medicine, gynecology, pediatrics, acupuncture and moxibustion, and especially excelled in surgery. *Mafeisan* (powder for anesthesia) developed by him was considered the earliest anesthetic in the history of world medicine and also opened up a new field for the expansion and development of surgery. His development was more than 1600 years earlier than ether anesthesia invented by dentist Moreton (1846).

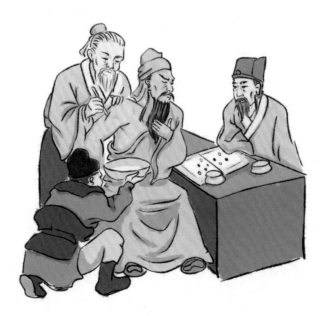

华佗还发明了"五禽戏",用来强身健体,预防疾病。华佗被害至今已1800多年了,但人们还永远怀念他,很多地方都有华佗的纪念场所。安徽亳州华祖庙里有一副对联,总结了华佗的一生:"医者刳腹,实别开岐圣门庭,谁知狱吏庸才,致使遗书归一炬;士贵洁身,岂屑侍奸雄左右,独憾史臣曲笔,反将厌事谤千秋。"

医圣张仲景

张仲景(150—219),名机,东汉南阳郡涅阳(今河南省南阳市邓州)人,东汉著名医学家。

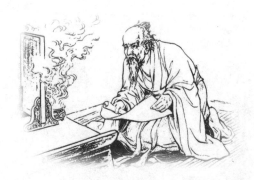

Hua Tuo also developed the wuqinxi (a set of physical exercises imitating the movements of the five animals), which can be practiced to tone up one's body and improve health and fitness. It has been more than 1,800 years since Hua Tuo was killed, but people have built some memorial sites to show their eternal remembrance. In the Huazu Temple located in Bozhou, Anhui province, there is a couplet inscribed summarizing Hua Tuo's whole life: "Hua Tuo created a new medical branch by opening patients' bellies to treat them. When he was imprisoned, Huo Tuo intended to entrust his medical book to a police officer, but the officer was so stupid and cowardly that he refused to keep the book. As a result, the book was burnt in the fire. What a shame! With strong moral principles and a noble mind, Hua Tuo despised serving the evil men around them. The only regret is that the official historians distorted the fact and defamed the legendary doctor Hua Tuo."

Zhang Zhongjing China's Medical Saint

Zhang Zhongjing (150-219 AD), whose courtesy name was Ji, was a famous physician born in Nieyang, Nanyang prefecture (now Dengzhou, Nanyang city, Henan province) in the Eastern Han.

张仲景出生于官宦世家，但是他立志行医，曾在长沙当太守时在大堂上为百姓看病，后来博采众方，著《伤寒杂病论》。该书确立了中医学"辨证论治"的规律，奠定了中医治疗学的基础，是中国最早的一部理法方药具备的经典著作，对后世有着深远的影响。因此，历代医家无不尊张仲景为"医圣"，故有"医圣者，即医中之尧舜也，荣膺此誉者，唯仲景先师。"《伤寒论》至今仍指导着临床实践，也是医家必读。

针灸鼻祖皇甫谧

皇甫谧(mì)(215—282)，字士安，自号玄晏先生。安定郡朝那县(今甘肃省灵台县)人，后徙居新安(今河南新安县)。三国西晋时期著名学者、医学家、史学家。

Born in an official family, Zhang Zhongjing aspired to a medical career. He once made diagnoses and gave treatment in the court when he held an official position in Changsha. He gathered a large collection of prescriptions, and wrote the *Shanghan Zabing Lun* (*Treatise on Exogenous Febrile and Miscellaneous Diseases*). The book, as the earliest classic combining theory, method, prescription with medication, established the law of syndrome differentiation and treatment in TCM, laid a foundation of TCM therapeutics and has exerted a far-reaching impact on later generations. Therefore, all physicians in the successive dynasties respected Zhang Zhongjing as China's medical saint. The following statement explains how exalted that title is: China's medical saint in the field of medicine is equivalent to the monarchs Yao and Shun in ancient China and Zhang Zhongjing was the only one who deserved this supreme honor. The *Shanghan Lun* (*Treatise on Exogenous Febrile Diseases*) still guides clinical practice and ranks among must-reads for TCM physicians.

Huangfu Mi The Originator of Acupuncture

Huangfu Mi (215-282 AD), whose courtesy name was Shi'an and who called himself Xuanyan, was born in Chaona county, Anding prefecture (now Lingtai county, Gansu Province), and later moved to Xin'an (now Xin'an county, Henan province). He was a famous scholar, physician and historian in the Three Kingdoms and the Western Jin.

他一生以著述为业，后得风痹（半身不遂），犹手不释卷。晋武帝时朝廷多次征召他入朝为官，都推辞不去。其著作《针灸甲乙经》是中国第一部针灸学的专著，在针灸学史上占有很高的学术地位，他因此被誉为"针灸鼻祖"。除此之外，他还编撰了《历代帝王世纪》《高士传》《逸士传》《列女传》《元晏先生集》等书，在医学史和文学史上都负有盛名。

药王孙思邈

孙思邈（541—682），京兆华原（今陕西省铜川市耀州区）人，他是中国乃至世界历史上著名的医学家和药物学家，被人们尊为"药王"。

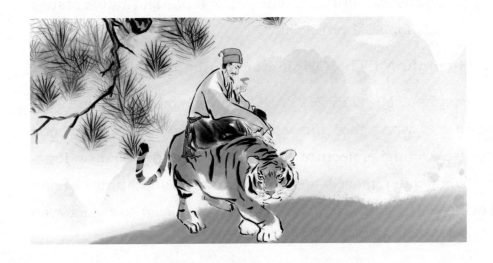

Huangfu Mi took writing as his lifelong career. Unfortunately, he suffered from wind impediment (hemiplegia) in his later years so that he immersed himself in reading. During the reign of Emperor Wudi of the Jin, the court invited him to be an official more than once, but he refused the invitations. The book *Zhenjiu Jiayi Jing* (*A-B Classic of Acupuncture and Moxibustion*) written by him is the first monograph on acupuncture and moxibustion in China and enjoys a high academic status in the field. Therefore, he has been hailed as the originator of acupuncture and moxibustion for his extraordinary achievements. In addition, he compiled a collection of books such as the *Lidai Diwang Shi Ji* (*Chronological Records of Emperors and Kings*), *Gaoshi Zhuan* (*Stories of the Brilliant Reclusive Scholars*), *Yi Shi Zhuan* (*Stories of Noble Reclusive Scholars*), *Lie Nü Zhuan* (*Stories of Great Women*) and *Yuan Yan Xiansheng Ji* (*Works of Yuan Yan*) and earned a great reputation in the history of medicine as well as literature.

Sun Simiao China's King of Medicine

Sun Simiao (541-682 AD), a native of Huayuan, Jingzhao (now Yaozhou, Tongchuan city, Shaanxi province), was a well-known physician and pharmacologist in the history of China and even the world, having been honored as China's king of medicine (an expert on herbalism) in history.

孙思邈不仅精于内科,而且擅长妇科、儿科、外科、五官科。在中医学上首次主张治疗妇女儿童疾病要单独设科,并在著作中首先论述妇、儿医学,声明是"崇本之义"。他从理论到实践,再由实践经验中提炼出新的医药学研究成果,以毕生精力撰写了医学著作《千金要方》和《千金翼方》。

孙思邈最为人称道的是医德,他提倡对患者一视同仁"皆如至尊","华夷愚智,普同一等"。他身体力行,一心赴救,不慕名利,用毕生精力实现了自己的医德思想。孙思邈的名著《千金要方》中,也把"大医精诚"的医德规范放在了极其重要的位置上来专门立题,重点讨论。

Sun Simiao was good at not only internal medicine, but also gynecology, pediatrics, surgery and facial features (otorhinolaryngology). In TCM, he was the first to advocate that a separate department should be set up for the treatment of women's and children's diseases, and also the first to discuss gynecology and pediatrics in his works, declaring that as the adhering to the fundamental. Having put theory into practice, he refined new medical research results from practical experience, and devoted all his life to writing medical works such as the *Qianjin Yao Fang* (*Invaluable Prescriptions*) and *Qianjin Yi Fang* (*A Supplement to Invaluable Prescriptions*).

Sun Simiao deserved the highest praise for his medical ethics. He treated patients equally, advocating all patients should be respected, whether Chinese or barbarians, foolish or wise, and they all are equal in my eyes. Practicing what he advocated, he devoted himself to saving people and never admired and courted fame and wealth. And he also practiced his medical ethics with all his life. In his book *Qianjin Yao Fang*, he also put the medical ethics of a master physician in an extremely important position and conducted a discussion.

药圣李时珍

李时珍(1518—1593),字东璧,晚年自号濒湖山人,湖北蕲州(今湖北省蕲春县蕲州)人,是中国明代著名的医学家、药理学家和博物学家,著有《本草纲目》《濒湖脉学》《奇经八脉考》等。

李时珍最著名的作品是《本草纲目》,这是一部详尽的医药学著作,共收录了1892种药物,包括植物药、动物药和矿物药,并详细描述了它们的性质、用途和制备方法。

李时珍在完成这部巨著时,进行了大量的实地考察和药物试验,体现了科学实证的精神。他的工作不仅在中国,而且在全球医学和自然科学领域都具有重要地位。

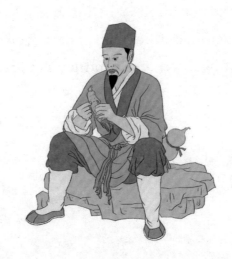

Li Shizhen China's Medicines Saint

Li Shizhen (1518-1593 AD), whose courtesy name was Dongbi and who called himself Binhu Shan Ren (a recluse living near Lake Binhu) in his twilight years, was a famous physician, pharmacologist, and naturalist, born in Qizhou, Hubei (now Qizhou, Qichun county, Hubei province) in the Ming dynasty. His main works include the *Bencao Gangmu* (*A Compendium of Materia Medica*), *Bin Hu Mai Xue* (*Binhu's Sphygmology*) and *Qi Jing Ba Mai Kao* (*Research on the Eight Extraordinary Meridians*).

Li Shizhen's most famous work is the *Bencao Gangmu*, an exhaustive medical and pharmacological work that lists 1, 892 types of substances from plants, animals and minerals, and provides detailed descriptions of their properties, functions, and preparation methods.

In completing this monumental work, Li Shizhen conducted extensive field research and pharmaceutical experiments, embodying the spirit of scientific empiricism. His contributions hold significant importance not only in China but also in the global fields of medicine and natural sciences.

第三章 中医药典籍

《黄帝内经》又称《内经》,是中国最早的典籍之一,也是中医学四大经典之首。作者并不是一人,而是由多种学术经验理论增补发展创作而来。冠以"黄帝"之名,意在溯源崇本,借以说明中国医药文化发祥之早,实非一时之言,亦非一人之手。

《黄帝内经》分《灵枢》和《素问》两部分。《素问》论述了医学理论、诊断方法、养生保健、治疗原则和哲学探讨;《灵枢》侧重于实际操作和治疗技术。《黄帝内经》奠定了人体生理、病理、诊断以及治疗的认识基础,是中国影响极大的一部医学著作,被称为医之始祖。

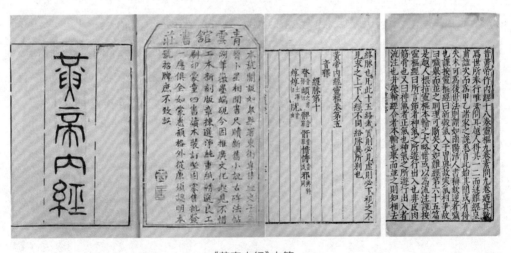

《黄帝内经》古籍

An Ancient Version of the *Huangdi Neijing* (*Huangdi's Classic of Medicine*)

Chapter 3 Classics of Traditional Chinese Medicine

The *Huangdi Neijing* (*Huangdi' s Classic of Medicine*), also known as the *Neijing*, is one of the earliest classics in China and tops four classics of Traditional Chinese Medicine (TCM). The book was not written by one single author, but a collection of the academic theories which supplemented and developed continuously. The name Huangdi was used to intend to trace back to the source and advocate the fundamentals of TCM culture, explaining how early TCM began. The book was not finished in one period and was not written by one author.

The *Huangdi Neijing* consists of two parts: *Lingshu* (*Miraculous Pivot*) and *Suwen* (*Basic Questions*). The *Suwen* discusses medical theories, diagnostic methods, health preservation, treatment principles, and philosophical exploration; the *Lingshu* focuses on practical operations and therapeutic techniques. The *Huangdi Neijing* laid a foundation for the understanding of human physiology, pathology, diagnosis and treatment, having been a medical work with enormous influence in China and known as the cornerstone of Traditional Chinese Medicine.

《难经》原名《黄帝八十一难经》，又称《八十一难》，是中医现存较早的经典著作。内容可能与秦越人（扁鹊）有一定关系。《难经》之"难"字，有"问难"或"疑难"之义。

全书采用问答方式，探讨和论述了中医的一些理论问题。其中，书中首创了独取寸口、寸关尺及浮中沉三部九候的切脉方法，脉证相参的辨证观，为中医脉学的发展做出了杰出贡献。在藏象学说方面，《难经》创立了命门学说，成为中医理论体系的重要组成部分。在经络学说方面，简明而系统地阐述了任脉、督脉、冲脉、带脉、阳维、阴维、阳跷、阴跷八条奇经的功能特点、循行路线、病变证候及其与十二正经的功能联系等，并总称之为"奇经八脉"。这一名称是《难经》最先提出的。

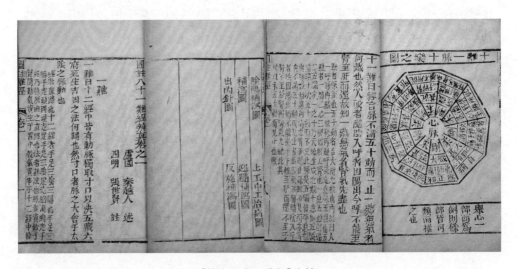

《黄帝八十一难经》古籍
An Ancient Version of the *Huangdi Ba Shi Yi Nan Jing*
(*Huangdi's Discussions on Eighty-one Difficult Issues*)

The *Nan Jing* (*Classic of Difficult Issues*), formerly known as the *Huangdi Ba Shi Yi Nan Jing* (*Huangdi's Discussions on Eighty-one Difficult Issues*) and also known as the *Ba Shi Yi Nan* (*Eighty-one Difficult Issues*), is an early classic of TCM. The content may have something to do with Qin Yueren (Bianque, a famous doctor in the Warring States period). The character "nan" in the Chinese name of the book means "questioning and arguing" or "difficulty".

The book discusses some theoretical problems of TCM in the form of question and answer. In the book, the authors initiated the pulse-feeling method of taking the cun, guan and chi pulse at three places with different degrees of strength and put forward the dialectical view of pulse and syndrome, which made outstanding contributions to the development of pulse science in TCM. In the theory of visceral manifestation, the *Nan Jing* developed the theory of gate of life and has become an important part of the theoretical system of TCM. In terms of meridian theory, the book concisely and systematically expounds on the functional characteristics, circulation routes, pathological changes and syndromes of the eight extraordinary meridians (ren, du, chong, dai, yangwei, yinwei, yangqiao and yinqiao) and their functional connections with the twelve meridians. The name of eight extraordinary meridians was first put forward in the *Nan Jing*.

　　《伤寒杂病论》是中医学著作之一,是中国中医院校开设的主要基础课程之一。《伤寒杂病论》系统地分析了伤寒的原因、症状、发展阶段和处理方法,创造性地把外感热性病的所有症状,归纳为六个证候群和八个辨证纲领,以六经来分析归纳疾病在发展过程中的演变和转归,以八纲来辨别疾病的属性、病位、邪正消长和病态表现。由于确立了分析病情、认识证候及临床治疗的法度,因此辨证论治不仅为诊疗外感热病提出了纲领性的法则,同时也给中医临床各科找出了诊疗的规律,成为指导后世医家临床实践的基本准绳。

　　《伤寒杂病论》是集秦汉以来中医药理论之大成,并广泛应用于中医医疗实践的专书,是中国医学史上影响最大的古典医著之一,也是中国第一部临床治疗学方面的巨著。

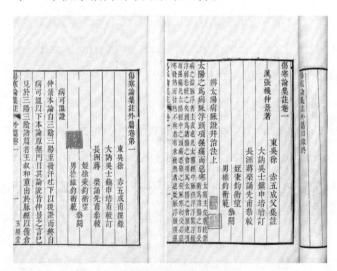

《伤寒杂病论》古籍

An Ancient Version of the *Shanghan Zabing Lun* (*Treatise on Exogenous Febrile and Miscellaneous Diseases*)

The *Shanghan Zabing Lun* (*Treatise on Exogenous Febrile and Miscellaneous Diseases*), is a classic of TCM and one of the major foundation courses offered by Chinese medical colleges and universities. It systematically analyzed the causes, symptoms, development stages and treatment methods of cold-induced diseases, creatively generalized all the symptoms of exogenous cold-induced diseases into six syndrome groups and eight syndrome differentiation guidelines, analyzed and summarized the evolution and conversion of diseases in the development process by six meridians, and identified the nature, location, waxing and waning of the evil and vital qi and morbid manifestations of diseases by eight principles. Syndrome differentiation and treatment set the standards for analyzing the state of a disease, identifying its syndromes and determining clinical treatment, so it not only put forward the programmatic rules for the diagnosis and treatment of all exogenous cold-induced diseases, but also figured out the rules of diagnosis and treatment for various clinical departments of TCM and provided the basic criteria for guiding the clinical practice of later physicians.

The *Shanghan Zabing Lun* captures the quintessence of medical theories originated since the Qin and Han dynasties and has been widely applied in medical practice. To some extent, it is one of the most influential classical medical works in the history of Chinese medicine and the first masterpiece of clinical therapeutics in China.

　　《神农本草经》又称《本草经》或《本经》,托名
"神农"所作,成书于汉代,是秦汉时期众多医学
家搜集、总结、整理当时药物学经验成果的专著,
是对中药学的第一次系统总结。

　　全书分三卷,载药365种,分上、中、下三品,
文字简练古朴,成为中药理论精髓。书中提出了
辨证用药的思想,所论药物适应病症有170多
种,对用药剂量、时间等都有具体规定,这也对中
药学起到了奠基作用。其中规定的大部分中药
学理论、配伍规则以及提出的"七情和合"原则,
一直在后世的用药实践中发挥重要作用,是中医
药物学理论发展的源头。此外,《神农本草经》中
对于药物的性味、产地与采制、炮制方法、服药方
法等都有涉及,极大地丰富了中药学的知识体
系。

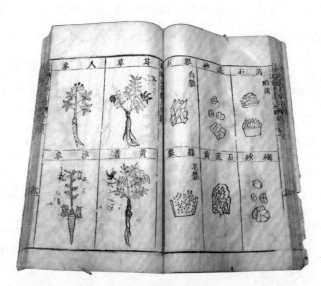

《神农本草经》古籍
An Ancient Version of the *Shennong Bencao Jing*
(*Shennong's Herbal*)

The *Shennong Bencao Jing* (*Shennong's Herbal*), also known as the *Classic of Herbal*, was written in the Han under the name of "Shennong". It is a treatise completed in the Qin and Han dynasties by many physicians who dedicated themselves to collecting, gathering up and summarizing the experience and achievements in pharmacology in their days, so it is regarded as the first systematic summary of TCM.

The book is divided into three volumes and records 365 kinds of medicinal materials which are classified into three grades: superior, medium and inferior. With its concise and unsophisticated words, it has been hailed as the theoretical essence of Chinese pharmacology. It also puts forward the idea of dialectical administration of medication. The medicinal materials discussed in the book can treat more than 170 diseases and the book contains specific provisions for the dosages and timing of medications, thus also playing a fundamental role in TCM. Most theories on Chinese pharmacology, combination rules and the seven principles of compatibility stipulated in the book have played a great role in the practice of medication and are thought of as the source of the development of the theories of Chinese pharmacology. In addition, the *Shennong Bencao Jing* touches upon the properties and flavors, growing areas, collecting and processing methods as well as administering methods, having greatly enriched the knowledge system of Chinese pharmacology.

第四章　中医药传承创新

在近现代中医药事业的发展进程中,中医药人始终肩负着传承创新的使命,努力推动中医药产业的现代化和国际化。屠呦呦和她发现的青蒿素就是中医药传承创新的典范。

屠呦呦的名字出自《诗经·小雅》中的"呦呦鹿鸣,食野之蒿"。"呦呦"是形容鹿的鸣叫;蒿,即青蒿,可当野菜食用,也是治疗疟疾的草药。疟疾,中国民间俗称"打摆子",是威胁人类生命的一大顽敌,全球每年约有4亿人次感染疟疾,主要集中在相对贫困的撒哈拉沙漠以南的非洲地区。20世纪60年代,由于疟原虫对金鸡纳碱类药物产生抗药性,全球100多个国家的2亿多疟疾患者面临无药可治的局面,死亡率急剧攀升。当时,中美两国都在开展抗疟研究,美方筛选了近30万种化合物却没有丝毫进展。

Chapter 4 Inheritance and Innovation of Traditional Chinese Medicine

In the development of Traditional Chinese Medicine (TCM) in modern and contemporary times, TCM practitioners have always borne the mission of inheritance and innovation, striving to promote the modernization and internationalization of the TCM industry. Tu Youyou, together with her discovery of artemisinin is a typical exemple of the inheritance and innovation of TCM.

Tu Youyou's given name Youyou comes from a line in the *Shi Jing, Xiao Ya* (*Classic of Poetry, Minor Odes*), "a herd of deer are bellowing and gazing wild Artemisia". "Youyou" refers to the cries of a deer. Artemisia, also called sweet wormwood, is an edible wild plant and is also used as herbal medicine to treat malaria. Malaria, commonly known as "teetering" in China, was a major threat to human life before artemisinin was discovered and used. About 400 million people worldwide are still infected with malaria every year, mainly in the relatively poor sub-Saharan Africa. In the 1960s, due to the resistance of malaria parasites to quinine drugs, more than 200 million malaria patients in more than 100 countries around the world were facing the situation of having no cure for malaria, and the mortality rate rose sharply. At that time, both China and the United States were conducting anti-malaria research, and the United States sifted out nearly 300,000 compounds but failed to make any further progress.

1969年，39岁的屠呦呦临危受命，被任命为“疟疾防治药物研究”项目中医研究院科研组长。通过翻阅历代本草医籍，四处走访老中医，甚至连相关信件都没放过，屠呦呦终于在2000多种方药中整理出一部含有640多种草药的《抗疟单验方集》，最终确定以青蒿为重点研究对象。可在最初的动物实验中，青蒿的效果并不明显，屠呦呦的研究也一度陷入僵局。

到底是哪个环节出了问题呢？屠呦呦再一次将注意力转向古老的中医学，重新在经典医籍中细细翻找。突然，葛洪所著《肘后备急方》中的几句话牢牢抓住了她的目光：“青蒿一握，以水二升渍，绞取汁，尽服之。”一语惊醒梦中人，屠呦呦马上意识到问题可能出在常用的“水煎”法上，因为高温会破坏青蒿中的有效成分，她随即另辟蹊径，采用低沸点溶剂进行实验。

葛仙翁肘後備急方卷之三
瘦樵程永培校
治寒熱諸瘧方第十六
治瘧病方鼠婦豆豉二七枚合搗令相和未發時服二丸欲發時服一丸
又方青蒿一握以水二升漬絞取汁盡服之
又方用獨父蒜於白炭上燒之末服方寸七
又方五月五日蒜一片去皮中破之刀割令容巴

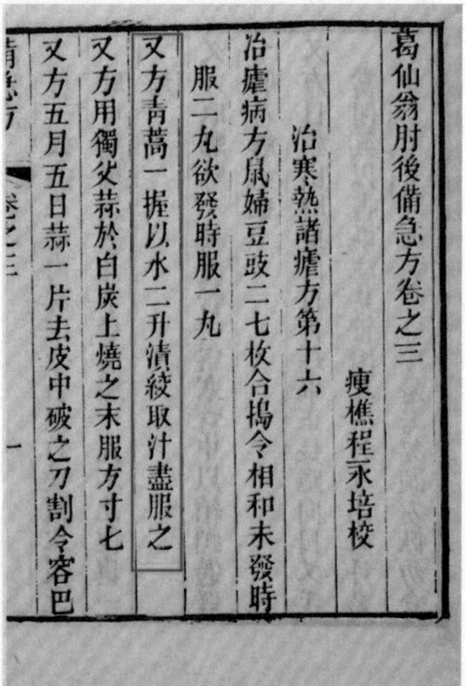

《肘后备急方》古籍
An Ancient Version of the *Zhouhou Beiji Fang* (*Handbook of Prescrptions for Emergencies*)

In 1969, 39-year-old Tu Youyou was appointed as a research team leader in charge of the project "Study on Medicines to Prevent and Cure Malaria" carried out by the Academy of TCM. By reading the medical books of past dynasties, visiting elderly doctors, and even reviewing relevant letters, Tu Youyou finally compiled the *Kang Nüe Dan Yanfang Ji* (*A Collection of Antimalarial Prescriptions*) containing more than 640 kinds of herbs from over 2000 prescriptions, she and her team finally focused on artemisinin. However, to her frustration, in the initial animal experiments, the effect of artemisinin was not significant, and Tu Youyou's research hit a deadlock.

Which step went wrong? Tu Youyou turned her attention to ancient TCM again and searched assiduously through its classics. Suddenly, a few words in Ge Hong's *Zhouhou Beiji Fang* (*Handbook of Prescrptions for Emergencies*) caught her eyes: "Take a handful of Artemisia annua, soak it in two liters of water, then squeeze out the juice, and take it all. " Tu's mind was awakened by the prescription and she immediately realized that the problem might lie in the commonly used decocting method, by which high temperature would destroy the active ingredients in Artemisia annua. Thus enlightened, she immediately found a new way to try low boiling point solvents in her experiments.

1971年,屠呦呦课题组在经过190次失败之后,终于在实验中发现了抗疟效果为100%的青蒿提取物。1972年,研究人员从这一提取物中提炼出抗疟有效成分青蒿素。青蒿素被世界公认为抗疟药物研究史上的新突破,也是中国第一个被世界公认的原始创新药物。

青蒿素能迅速消灭人体内的疟原虫,与其他抗疟药物相比,青蒿素类药物不良反应轻微、治愈率高且价格便宜,被许多非洲民众称为"中国神药"。自问世以来,全球数亿人因此受益。坦桑尼亚、赞比亚等非洲国家近年来疟疾死亡率显著下降,一个重要原因就是广泛使用青蒿素复方药物。

2004年5月,世界卫生组织正式将青蒿素复方药物列为治疗疟疾的首选药物。世界权威医学刊物《柳叶刀》的统计显示,青蒿素复方药物对恶性疟疾的治愈率达到97%。据此,世卫组织当年就要求在疟疾高发的非洲地区采购和分发100万剂青蒿素复方药物。

In 1971, having suffered 190 failures, Tu's team discovered Artemisia annua extract with 100% anti-malarial effect in the 191st experiment. In 1972, researchers extracted artemisinin, an effective anti-malarial ingredient, from the extract. Artemisinin now has been recognized by the whole world as a new breakthrough in the history of anti-malarial drug research as well as China's first originally innovative drug.

Artemisinin can quickly eliminate malaria parasites in the human body. Compared with other anti-malarial drugs, artemisinin drugs have milder adverse reactions, a higher cure rate and lower price, so it is called Chinese miracle drug by many African people. Since its advent, hundreds of millions of people around the world have benefited from it. One root cause of the dramatic decline of malaria mortality in Tanzania, Zambia and other African countries in recent years is the widespread distribution of artemisinin compound drugs.

In May 2004, World Health Organization (WHO) officially listed artemisinin compound drugs as the first choice for the treatment of malaria. Statistics from *The Lancet*, an authoritative medical journal, showed that the cure rate of artemisinin compound drugs for falciparum malaria is 97%. As a result, WHO requested that African regions where malaria is highly prevalent should purchase and distribute 1 million doses of artemisinin compound drugs.

2011年,因为发现治疗疟疾的青蒿素,挽救了全球,特别是发展中国家的数百万人的生命,屠呦呦获得美国拉斯克临床医学奖。2015年,屠呦呦等三位科学家被授予诺贝尔生理学或医学奖,这是中国医学界迄今为止获得的最高奖项,也是中医药成果获得的最高奖项。2019年9月,国家主席习近平签署主席令,授予屠呦呦"共和国勋章"。

青蒿素被誉为传统中医药献给世界的礼物,是中医药学为世界人民的健康福祉做出的重大贡献,也标志着中医药的研究得到了国际科学界的高度关注。青蒿素的故事再次表明:中国医药学是一个伟大的宝库,应当努力发掘,加以传承创新。

In 2011, Tu Youyou won the Lasker Prize for Clinical Medicine in the United States for discovering malaria-curing artemisinin, which saved millions of lives around the world, especially in developing countries. In 2015, the Nobel Prize in Physiology or Medicine was awarded to Tu and two other scientists. The award is the highest award to Chinese medical practitioners so far and the highest award won by any achievement in TCM. In September 2019, President Xi Jinping signed a presidential decree to award Tu a Medal of the Republic.

Artemisinin is praised as a gift from TCM to the whole world as well as an extraordinary contribution made by TCM to the health and well-being of the people around the globe. Its approval indicates that the research on TCM has received high attention from the international scientific community. The story of artemisinin once again shows that Chinese medicine is a great treasure house to be explored, inherited and innovated.

第五章　中医药走向世界

只有民族的,才是世界的。中医药作为中华民族的国粹,不但为中华民族的繁衍生息做出了巨大的贡献,也对世界文明的进步产生了深远的影响。

中医药的海外传播最早可追溯到秦汉时期以前,隋唐时期开始逐渐体系化、规范化,至宋金元时期中药、针灸等已作为完整的系统向海外传播。早期的传播路径主要有古代丝绸之路和海上丝绸之路,影响力由近及远依次递减。在16—18世纪,欧洲人开始接触中医,此时的中医主要由学习了中医的日本医生及欧洲传教士传入。近代以来,随着国际交往的深入和华人向世界各地流动,中医药特别是针灸在国外的传播明显增加。古代丝绸之路中医药输出的方式,除外交赠送、军事战争等特殊情况外,主要还是依靠贸易和移民。而影响传播的因素则包括宗教、文化、军事、政治、经济、科技等方面。

Chapter 5 Chinese Medicine Going Golbal

What is truly national belongs to the world. Traditional Chinese Medicine (TCM), as the quintessence of the Chinese nation, has not only made great contributions to the reproduction of the Chinese nation, but also has a far-reaching impact upon the progress of world civilization.

The overseas spread of TCM can be traced back to the Qin and Han dynasties, and it started to be systematized and standardized in the Sui and Tang dynasties. By the Song, Jin and Yuan, TCM, including acupuncture and moxibustion, had been spread abroad as a complete system. The early propagation paths mainly included the ancient Silk Road and maritime Silk Road routes, and their influence decreased from the near to the distant places. Between the 16th and 18th centuries, Europeans began to learn about TCM, which was mainly introduced by Japanese doctors and European missionaries who had made a study of it. Since modern times, with the deepening of international exchanges and flow of the Chinese into all parts of the world, the spread of TCM, especially acupuncture and moxibustion, has increased significantly. Apart from serving as a diplomatic present, being introduced along with military conflicts and under other circumstances, the export of TCM along the ancient Silk Road mainly relied on trade and immigration. Other factors connected with the spread of TCM include religion, culture, military status, politics, economy, science and technology.

自20世纪70年代世界兴起针灸热之后，以欧美国家为主要方向、以针灸为先导、瞄准中医药国际标准，并致力于打入国际主流药品市场的中医药国际化发展策略，逐渐得到较为广泛的认同。

中医药"一带一路"建设为新形势下中医药走向世界提供了新的目标方向。作为国家"一带一路"倡议的重要内容和理想载体，中医药合作交流已经成为"一带一路"建设新的亮点，有着巨大的发展潜力。共建"一带一路"国家不仅具有相对更深的历史渊源，对中医药还有着现实的客观需求。在参与各方的共同努力下，中医药"一带一路"建设已经取得初步成效。中国各省（直辖市、自治区）"一带一路"中医药发展的思路举措、国外致力于中医药技术推广和推动中医药立法、中医药海外中心等平台的建设，都为中医药"一带一路"建设积累了宝贵的经验。

Since a craze of acupuncture and moxibustion—starting in European countries and America in the 1970s, TCM, with acupuncture and moxibustion as its forerunner, began to target the European countries and America and international standards of TCM began to be formulated. Meanwhile, TCM has been aiming at entering the international mainstream drug markets for a long time and has gradually been widely recognized.

The construction of the Belt and Road Initiative integrating TCM provides a new strategic direction for TCM to enter the world under the new situation. As an indispensable part and ideal carrier of the Belt and Road Initiative, TCM, with its cooperation and exchange between China and other countries, has become a new bright spot for the Belt and Road Initiative and has great potential for development. The countries co-construction the Belt and Road not only have relatively deeper historical relationship with China, but also have realistic and objective needs for TCM. With the joint efforts of all parties involved, the construction of the Belt and Road Initiative of TCM has achieved initial results. The developing ideas and measures of TCM in the frame of the Belt and Road Initiative in various provinces, municipalities directly under the Central Government and autonomous regions, the promotion of TCM abroad, the starting of TCM legislation, and the construction of overseas TCM centers have all accumulated valuable experience for the promotion of TCM in the general frame of the Belt and Road Initiative.

随着中医药现代化和国际化的步伐不断前行,相信中医药一定会成为中国走向世界的一张无比靓丽的名片,成为构建人类健康命运共同体的重要一环。

With its pace of modernization and internationalization, we believe that TCM will become an incomparably impressive business card for China to go into the world and an important part of building a global community of human health and shared destiny.

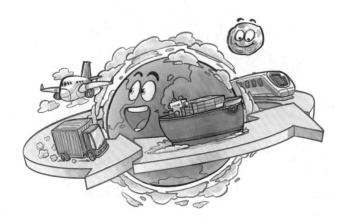

第二单元　中医药学蕴藏的智慧

中医药在历史发展进程中,兼收并蓄、创新开放,形成了独特的生命观、健康观、疾病观、防治观,蕴含和体现了中华民族深邃的哲学思想。中国的中医药一直为保障中华民族的健康及战胜人类疾病做贡献,中医药智慧也一直维系着中华民族上下五千年的繁衍,以致当今华夏大地成为拥有世界最多人口的泱泱大国。随着中医药走向现代化,我们确信中医药的大智慧,也必将造福于全人类。

Unit II The Wisdom of Traditional Chinese Medicine

In the process of its historical development, Traditional Chinese Medicine (TCM) has been inclusive and innovative, forming its unique concepts on life, health, disease, prevention and treatment, which embodies the profound philosophical ideas of the Chinese people. It has been contributing to the protection of the health of the Chinese people and to their victory over diseases, and maintaining the continuous and stable reproduction of the people for five thousand years. That is why today China has become a vast country with the largest population in the world. With the modernization of TCM, it is firmly convinced that the great wisdom contained in it will also benefit all other nations in the world.

这个单元将和大家讲述中医"天人合一"的整体观念和治未病的预防思想,介绍中医"辨证论治"的诊疗思维以及"阴阳五行学说",同时带领同学们从藏象学说、经络学说的角度来认识人体的生命现象和健康问题。让我们一起开启学习之旅,领略深邃的中医智慧。

This unit will tell the readers something about the holistic concept of harmony between man and nature in TCM and the preventive thought of prophylactic treatment of disease, introducing the diagnostic and therapeutic thinking of syndrome differentiation and treatment and the theories of yin-yang and five elements, which are proper to the medicine, and leading everyone to understand life phenomena and health problems of the human body from the perspective of the visceral manifestation and the meridian theory. Let's start our learning journey together and appreciate the inspiring wisdom of TCM.

第六章 中医的整体观念

　　《黄帝内经》是中国古代人民根据长时间生活实践所总结的第一部中医学巨著,该书认为,人体与自然界是密不可分的,自然界的变化随时影响着人体,人类在能动地适应自然和改造自然的过程中维持着正常的生命活动。这种机体自身整体性和内外环境统一性的思想即整体观念,也被称为"天人合一"。整体观念是中国古代唯物论和辩证思想在中医学中的体现。

　　中医学的整体观念强调人体内外环境的整体和谐、协调和统一,认为人体是一个有机整体,既强调人体内部环境的统一性,又注重人与外界环境的统一性。所谓外界环境是指人类赖以存在的自然和社会环境。

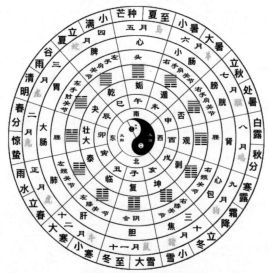

中医基础知识示意图
Diagram of Traditional Chinese Medicine
Basic Konwledge

Chapter 6 The Holistic Concept of Traditional Chinese Medicine

The Huangdi Neijing (*Huangdi's Classic of Medicine*), the first great work of Traditional Chinese Medicine (TCM) summarized by the ancient Chinese people on the basis of their long life practice, holds that the human body is inseparably linked to nature. Any change in nature at any moment affects the human body. Human beings maintain normal life activities in the process of trying actively to adapt to and transform nature. This idea that the human body itself is an integral system and that the internal and external environments are unified, is known as the holistic concept, also called the unity of man and nature in Chinese culture.

The holistic concept of TCM emphasizes the overall harmony, coordination and unity of the internal and external environments of the human body, holding that the human body is an organic whole, which not only attaches importance to the unity of the internal environment of the human body, but also pays attention to the unity of the human body and its external environment. The latter refers to the natural and social environment on which human beings are dependent.

中医学根据朴素的唯物主义"天人一气"的"天人合一"说,用医学、天文学、气象学等自然科学材料,论证并丰富了"天人合一"说,提出了"人与天地相参"(《素问·咳论》)的"天人一体"观,强调"善言天者,必有验于人"(《素问·举痛论》),把人的需要和对人的研究放在天人关系理论的中心位置。

中医学的"天人合一"观强调人与自然的和谐一致。人和自然有着共同的规律,人的生长壮老已受自然规律的制约,人的生理病理也随着自然的变化而产生相应的变化。人应通过养生等手段,积极主动地适应自然。

顺应自然,即人体要顺应自然规律,才能维持正常的生命活动。要做到天人相应,就要以大自然的变化规律为起居活动的准则,使我们的日常生活符合养生的要求。比如夏天天气炎热,吃的食物就不要太热了。

Based on the simple materialist ideas of unity of man and nature in qi and harmony between man and nature, TCM further illuminated and enriched the theory of "harmony between man and nature" with scientific facts from medicine, astronomy and meteorology, putting forward the holistic concept that "man is one with heaven and earth", stressing that "those who know how to speak about heaven must get such experience from studying man". From these we can see that the needs and study of human beings are always in the central part of the theory of the relationship between heaven and man in TCM.

The concept of harmony between man and nature in TCM emphasizes a harmonious relationship between man and nature. Man and nature share common laws. Human growth and aging are subject to the laws of nature, and human physiology and pathology change accordingly with the changes of nature. People should actively adapt to nature through health preservation and other health-caring means.

Compliance with nature means that the human body has to go with the laws of nature to maintain normal life activities. In order to achieve the harmony between man and nature, it is necessary to adopt the basic laws of change in nature as the rules of rising and resting regularly and ensure that our daily life meets the requirements of good health. For example, in summer, it is not advisable to eat food that is too hot.

饮食有节，即饮食要适度。如果暴饮暴食；或者饮食无规律，饥一顿饱一顿；或者偏食挑食，都会损伤身体。

起居有常，就是指我们日常生活各个方面都要有一定的规律。如果生活无规律，不善于保养，就会损害身体的健康。

Eating and drinking in moderation means that we shouldn't eat or drink too much. It is harmful to our health to eat or drink excessively or irregularly, or be partial to particular kinds of food or particular about food.

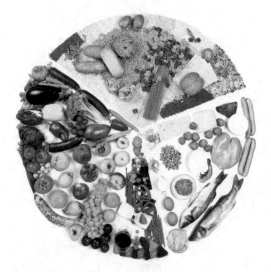

Rising and resting regularly means that we should follow regular patterns of going to bed and getting up, as well as of other aspects of our daily life. If our activities are irregular and damaging, our health will be failing.

第七章 中医药的预防观念

春秋时期有位名医叫扁鹊,有一次去见蔡桓公。他认真看了一会儿,对桓公说:"你有病了,要赶快医治,否则病情将会加重!"桓公听了笑着说:"我没有病。"十天以后,扁鹊又去见桓公,说他的病已经加重,如果不治,还会加重。桓公不理睬他。再过了十天,扁鹊又去见桓公,说他的病已经很严重了,再不从速医治,就会有生命危险。桓公仍旧不理睬他。又过了十天,扁鹊去见桓公时,对他望了一望,转身就走。

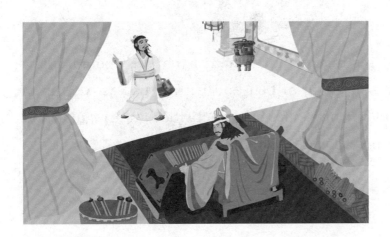

桓公觉得很奇怪,派人去问扁鹊。扁鹊说:"刚开始发病时,只要用熏蒸发热就能治疗;病到了肌肤之中,用针灸砭石可以治疗;疾病深入到肠胃,要用猛药重剂才能治愈;病若是到了骨髓里,那就没有办法救治了。"五天以后,桓公浑身疼痛,派人去请扁鹊,扁鹊却早已经逃到秦国了,桓公不久就死掉了。

Chapter 7 The Prophylactic Concept of Traditional Chinese Medicine

During the Spring and Autumn period, a famous doctor named Bianque went to visit king Cai Huangong. Bianque looked at him carefully for a while and said to the king, "You are ill. You must be cured quickly, otherwise your illness will get worse!" Hearing this, Cai Huangong smiled and remarked, "I am not ill at all." Ten days later, Bianque went to see the king again and said that his illness had worsened and would get even worse if he did not get cured. Cai Huangong ignored his warning. Ten days later, Bianque went to see the king once again and said that his illness was already very serious, and if he did not receive immediate treatment, his life would be in danger. Cai Huangong still ignored his warning. Another ten days later, Bianque went to see the king. He looked at Cai Huangong for a while, then turned and left.

The king felt very strange and sent one of his men to ask Bianque about it. Bianque replied, "At the beginning of the illness, it could be instantly cured only by fuming and steaming the patient; when the illness reached the skin, it could be cured with stone needles; when the illness reached the stomach and intestines, it could be cured only in large doses of powerful medicine; when the illness reached the bone marrow, there could be no cure any longer." Five days later, the king felt sore all over and sent for the doctor, but he had already fled to the Qin state. Cai Huangong died soon afterwards.

这个故事启示我们,疾病要重在预防,等到疾病发生发展之后,可能会延误治疗的最佳时机。这很好地体现了中医"治未病"思想。

中医"治未病"体现了中国传统文化中"未雨绸缪""防患于未然"的预防理念。《黄帝内经》所说:"上工治未病,不治已病,此之谓也。"就是说高明的大夫,会提前调理预防未来可能发生的疾病,防止疾病的发生发展。其主要思想是未病先防和既病防变。

未病先防就是在没有发病之前,做好各种预防工作,以防止疾病的发生。中医学在长期和疾病作斗争的实践中,积累了丰富的有关预防疾病的方法。如调养精神情志、适应四时气候、加强身体锻炼、注意饮食起居等,都对疾病的预防起着很重要的作用。

The story tells us that prevention is better than cure. Treatment is already late when a disease has already developed. This is a good example of the preventive treatment of diseases in Traditional Chinese Medicine (TCM).

The idea of "preventive treatment of diseases" in TCM embodies the preventive concept of "preparing for a rainy day" or "preventing something before it happens" in traditional Chinese culture. " The preventive treatment of disease" is derived from the quotation in *Huangdi Neijing* (*Huangdi's Classic of Medicine*): "The superior practitioner initiates a cure where there is no disease yet, he does not cure where there is already a disease, that is what is meant here." This tells us that a great doctor is able to take appropriate measures to prevent the occurrence and progress of a disease, and prevent a disease that is likely to begin. The gist is prevention of a disease occurring and prevention of a disease progressing.

Prevention of a disease occurring is to take a variety of measures before the onset of a disease to prevent its occurrence. In the long practice of fighting against diseases, TCM has accumulated various methods with regard to prevention. The methods, such as regulating the spirit and emotion, adapting to seasonal changes, keeping fit through regular exercise, eating and drinking properly, rising and resting regularly, etc., have been playing a very important role in preventing diseases before they occur.

既病防变,就是已经得了病之后要防止疾病的变化。所以,疾病发生后,就应该早期诊断、早期治疗,以防止疾病的发展。只有及时诊治,才能避免疾病步步深入,控制或减少疾病的恶化,收到良好的治疗效果。

每年进入夏季的三伏天,同学们就会看到中医医院的门诊大厅里挤满了进行贴敷治疗的人。三伏贴是根据中医"冬病夏治"的原理来实施的一种治未病的方法。"冬病"是指一些好发于冬季或者遇寒冷天气容易加重的疾病。"夏治"是指在夏季三伏天,一年中最热、阳气最旺的时候,通过各种中医治疗措施,达到治疗或者预防"冬病"的目的。冬病夏治的方法有很多,其中最具代表性的就是三伏贴。

Prevention of a disease progressing is to prevent the likely bad progression of the disease after it has already occurred. Therefore, after the occurrence of a disease, early diagnosis and early treatment are necessary to prevent the disease from getting worse. Only timely diagnosis and treatment can avoid the progression of the disease, control or slow the worsening of the disease, or bring about remarkable curative effects.

Every year in the dog days of summer, we very often see hospitals of TCM crowded with people for treatment with applications or skin patches. Wearing a dog-day patch is a method of preventive treatment based on the principle of "treating winter diseases in summer" in TCM. A "winter disease" refers to one that is likely to occur in winter or aggravate in cold weather. "Summer treatment" refers to `the treatment or prevention of a "winter disease" by TCM measures during the dog days of summer, or the sunniest and hottest days of the year. There are many ways to treat winter diseases in summer, among which the most representative is with dog-day patches.

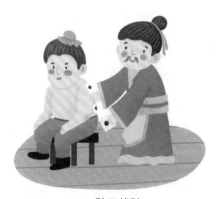

贴三伏贴
Wear a Dog-day Patch

第八章 中医药的诊疗理念

三国时期,倪寻和李延病了,一同到名医华佗那儿看病。两人都是头疼,全身发热。华佗仔细诊断后,却给他们开出了不同的药方。两人非常好奇:"我们病情一样,吃的药为什么有那么大的区别?"

华佗看出了他们的疑问,问道:"生病前你们都做了什么?"倪寻回忆说:"我昨天赴宴回来,就感到有点不舒服,今天就头疼发烧了。"

"我好像是昨天没盖好被子受凉了。"李延答道。

"那就对了。"华佗解释,"倪寻是因为昨天饮食不洁,内部伤食引起的头疼身热,应该通肠胃,所以我给你开了泻下的药;而李延是因为外感风寒引起的感冒发烧,应该吃发汗的药。病情表面差不多,但你们得病的原因不同,治疗的办法也会不同。"

Chapter 8 The Diagnosis & Treatment Concept of Traditional Chinese Medicine

During the Three Kingdoms period, Ni Xun and Li Yan fell ill and went together to see the miracle doctor Hua Tuo. Both of them had a headache and were burning up. After a careful examination, Hua Tuo gave them different prescriptions. The two men were so extremely curious, "We have the same illness, but why are our medicines quite different?"

Hua Tuo noticed that they doubted about their medicines and asked, "What happened before you got sick?" Ni Xun replied, "I came back from a banquet yesterday and felt a little sick, but today, I have had a headache and fever."

"I got a cold last night, I think. I failed to cover myself up." Li Yan replied.

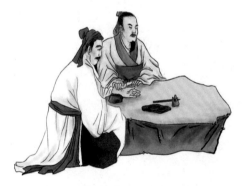

"That's it" Hua Tuo explained, "Ni Xun is suffering from a headache and fever because of bad food of yesterday, so I gave some medicine for diarrhea. Li Yan is suffering from a cold and fever because he had a cold. So some medicine for sweating should be effective. Your symptoms are similar, but the causes and treatments are different.

　　倪、李二人觉得华佗说得非常有道理,回去吃下不同的药,第二天,两人的病就好了。后世就用"对症下药"来形容针对事物的问题所在,采取有效的措施。

　　"对症下药"所体现的中医智慧,就是中医最具特色的诊断和治疗方法——辨证论治。这是中医认识疾病和治疗疾病的基本原则,是中医学对疾病的一种特殊的研究和处理方法。辨证论治突出了个性化的中医思路,强调以人为本。

The two men thought what Hua Tuo said was reasonable. They went back to take their own medicine respectively. The next day, they fully recovered. Since then, the idiom "prescribing the right medicine for an illness" has been used to describe a situation where the correct action has to be taken to solve a certain problem.

The wisdom embodied by the idiom is the most distinctive method of diagnosis and treatment of Traditional Chinese Medicine (TCM) —treatment based on syndrome differentiation. It is a basic principle of identifying and treating diseases, and also a special perspective of understanding and dealing with diseases. The method highlights the individualized way adopted by TCM, emphasizing that patients are treated differently, that is, different treatments need to be given to patients individually based on their specific conditions.

　　辨证和论治,是诊治疾病过程中相互联系不可分割的两个方面,是理论和实践相结合的体现,是理法方药在临床上的具体运用,是指导中医临床的基本原则。辨证,就是将四诊(望、闻、问、切)所收集的资料,如症状和体征(如脉象、舌象),通过分析、综合,辨清疾病的原因、性质、部位,以及邪正之间的关系,加以概括、判断为某种性质的证。论治,又称施治,则是根据辨证的结果,确定相应的治疗方法。辩证是论治的基础,辩证不准确,则会导致出现南辕北辙的严重后果。

　　望诊,是医生运用视觉观察患者全身和局部的一切可见征象(如精神状态、面色、皮肤、指甲、舌象等)、排出物及分泌物,以了解健康或疾病的状态。比如,扁鹊见蔡桓公的故事中,就阐述了扁鹊通过"望诊"的方法发现蔡桓公的疾病。

As the two interrelated and inseparable aspects of diagnosis and treatment, syndrome differentiation and treatment determination embodies a combination of theory and practice, and a practical and clinical application of theories, methods, formulas and medicinals. Thus, it is constantly considered a basic principle guiding the clinical practice of TCM. The syndrome differentiation refers to the analysis and assessment of symptoms and signs (such as pulse conditions and tongue coating) collected by the four diagnostic methods (observing, listening and smelling, inquring, and pulse-taking) to determine the cause, nature, and location of the disease and the relationship between the pathogenic factors and the healthy factors for classifying the data as a particular syndrome with certain characteristics. The treatment determination, which actually means deciding or giving medical treatment, is based on the results of syndrome differentiation to determine the appropriate treatment. Differentiation is the first step, and an inaccurate differentiation certainly leads to a wrong treatment.

Observing, or visual diagnosis, is a doctor's observation of all visible forms or manifestations (such as mental state, complexion, skin, nails, tongue coating, etc.), excretions such as sputum, urine and stool, etc., and secretions of the whole body or parts of the body, in order to get to know the physical and mental state of a patient. For example, in the story of the renowned doctor Bianque (407-310 BC) meeting with king Cai Huangong, it is recorded that Bianque discovered the disease of Cai Huangong just by observing.

闻诊,是医生通过听觉听声音和通过嗅觉闻气味,以了解病体发出的各种异常声音和气味,诊察病情。

问诊,是通过询问患者或陪诊者,了解疾病的发生、发展、治疗经过、症状及其他与疾病有关的情况,以诊察疾病的方法。

切诊,包括脉诊和按诊两部分内容。脉诊是按脉搏,按诊是在患者身躯上一定的部位触摸、按压,以了解疾病的内在变化或体表反应。

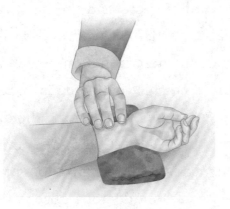

脉诊
Diagnosis by Feeling the Pulse

中医学在历史上所形成的辨证分类方法有很多种,其中最基本的方法就是八纲辨证。八纲是辨证的总纲,包括阴、阳、表、里、寒、热、虚、实。八纲辨证就是运用八纲通过四诊所掌握的各种临床资料进行分析综合,以辨别病变的部位、性质、邪正盛衰及病症类别等情况,以便对症下药。

Listening and smelling is that a doctor of TCM is able to diagnose a patient by various abnormal sounds and smells from his or her body and determine what he or she is suffering from.

Asking or inquiring is a method of diagnosing diseases by asking patients or those accompanying them questions to know about the occurrence, development, previous treatment, symptoms, as well as any other disease-related information.

Pulse diagnosis consists of two aspects: taking the pulse and palpating parts of the body. Pulse diagnosis is taking or feeling the pulse, while palpating is touching or pressing the affected parts of the patient's body to make sure of the adverse changes inside the body or on the surface of the body.

In the history of TCM, there have been several classifications of syndrome differentiation, among which the most basic is the eight principles, which includs yin and yang, exterior and interior, cold and heat, and deficiency and excess. The eight-principle differentiation is to analyze and synthesize various clinical data collected by the four diagnostic methods, so as to determine the location, nature, and severity of a certain disease, and thus to give the right prescription for the disease.

第九章 中医的阴阳五行学说

阴阳五行学说是中国传统文化的重要理念，后来中医学家在长期医疗实践的过程中将这些学说应用到了医学上来，用以说明人类生命起源、生命现象、病理现象，帮助临床医生更好地诊断和治疗疾病，成为中医学理论的重要组成部分，对中医学理论体系的形成和发展发挥了重要作用。

中医学认为，世间万物都是对立统一的，一为阳，一为阴。如上为阳、下为阴，外为阳、内为阴，热为阳、寒为阴，气为阳，血为阴。阴阳这两大势力相互对立，又相互依存。二者之间相互影响。

Chapter 9 The Theories of Yin-Yang & Five Elements in Traditional Chinese Medicine

The theories of yin-yang and five elements are fundamental concepts of traditional Chinese culture. In long medical practice, practitioners of Traditional Chinese Medicine (TCM) applied the theories to medicine to explain the origin of human life, physiological and pathological phenomena, and help clinicians better diagnose and treat diseases. Therefore, they have become an important part of TCM and played a considerable role in the formation and development of the theorical system of TCM.

According to TCM, everything in the world is the unity of opposites: one being yang and the other yin. For example, the upper is yang while the lower is yin, the external is yang while the internal is yin, heat is yang while cold is yin, qi is yang while blood is yin. The two forces are both opposed to each other and depend on each other. The two influence each other.

　　所谓五行,就是金、木、水、火、土。所谓"金"并不是黄金,"水"亦不是和杯中喝的水一样,千万不要认为五行就是五种物质。根据五行学说,"木曰曲直",凡是具有生长、升发、条达舒畅等作用或性质的事物,均归属于木;"火曰炎上",凡具有温热、升腾作用的事物,均归属于火;"土爰稼穑",凡具有生化、承载、受纳作用的事物,均归属于土;"金曰从革",凡具有清洁、肃降、收敛等作用的事物则归属于金;"水曰润下",凡具有寒凉、滋润、向下运动的事物则归属于水。

　　五行学说认为,五行之间存在着生、克、乘、侮的关系。五行的相生相克关系可以解释事物之间的相互联系,而五行的相乘相侮则可以用来表示事物之间平衡被打破后的相互影响。

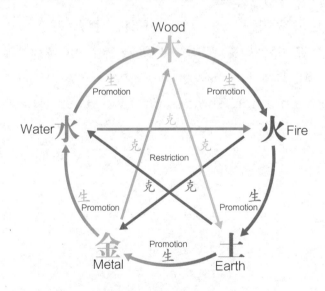

五行相生相克关系示意图
Schematic Diagram of the Laws of Promtion and Restriction Among the Five Elements

The five elements refer to metal, wood, water, fire and earth, as well as their motions and changes in the natural world. The word "metal" does not really mean a metal, and "water" is not the same as the water in your cup. Therefore, the elements are closely related and reflect the seasonal changes those early thinkers saw in the world around them. According to the theory, "wood bends and strengthens", which means the stem and branches can bend, strengthen, and grow upward and outward, so all things with such functions or properties are attributed to wood; "fire burns and flares up", which means fire is characterized by warmth, heat and going up. By extension of its meaning, anything with such functions is attributed to fire; "earth provides for sowing and reaping", which means that earth is for farming, or all things with the functions or properties of generation, holding and receiving are attributed to earth; "metal works for change", which originally means metal takes shape based on change, and so, metaphorically, things with the functions of clearing, falling and contracting are attributed to gold; "water moistens and flows downward", which means water has the properties of moistening and moving downward, and thus anything with the functions of being cold or cool, moistening and going downward is attributed to water.

Among the five elements, there is a relationship of mutual promotion, restriction, subjugation and violation. The inter-promotion and inter-restriction can explain the inter-connection between things, while the inter-subjugation and inter-violation can be used to express the mutual influence between things after the balance is broken.

　　阴阳五行学说是中医药学的核心理论，贯穿于整个中医理论体系和临床治疗体系之中，可以应用于中医学对藏象、经络、病因、病机、诊法、治则、药理等各个方面的认识，对于中医药学的建立具有重要的指导作用。

The theories of yin-yang and five elements, the core theories of TCM, runs through the whole system of Chinese medical theories and clinical treatment and plays a key role in the establishment of TCM. Thus, the theories are helpful in understanding basic concepts of TCM, like manifestations of organs, symptoms, channels and collaterals, etiology, pathogenesis, diagnostic methods, treatment principle and pharmacology, etc.

第十章 神奇的经络

中医学的发展除了深受古代科学技术、社会文化、古代哲学思想的影响之外,更主要的是古人有大量的医学实践。这其中就包括最为原始和简单的解剖活动,而这也是有明确的文献记载可以证实的。在原始的解剖活动中,医家们就发现人体内有很多管道,这些管道纵横交错,分布在人体的各个地方。古人联系对自然界河流湖泊的感性认识,形成了对经络的初步认识。

故而对经络基本功能的认识也是依据对自然界河流湖泊的感性认识,人体内的这些管道就像大地上的河流,有明确的主干,也有细小的分支。所以将人体中的主干管道称为"经脉",将联络主干的细小分支则称为"络脉",而经络就是经脉和络脉的总称。

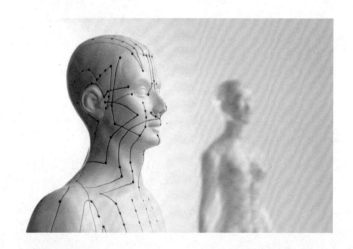

Chapter 10 Magical Meridians & Collaterals

The development of Traditional Chinese Medicine (TCM) has not only been deeply influenced by ancient sciences and technology, social culture and ancient philosophy, also by a large amount of medical practice in ancient times. The practice includes the most primitive and simple anatomical activities, which can be confirmed today by clear documentation. Through primitive anatomical activities, physicians found that in the human body there are many channels, which crisscross and are distributed throughout the body. With this discovery, ancient people associated their first-hand knowledge of rivers and lakes in nature and developed the primary concept of meridians.

Therefore, the knowledge formed the basis for the theory of meridians. The channels in the body are like rivers on earth, some of which are main channels and some minor branches. The channels are called "meridians", while the branches connecting the channels called "collaterals", and the two put together are technically called "meridians and collaterals".

　　古人认为，人体特定部位间的联系是通过特定的经脉或络脉实现的，这种联系包括体表与体表之间、体表与脏腑之间的联系。经络系统就像交通运行系统，既有主干道，也有辅道，还有各种通道的分支。其中，经脉为主干通道，包括十二经脉和奇经八脉。络脉为辅助通道，包括十五络脉、十二经筋、十二皮部等。孙络和浮络就是通道分支，各个穴位就是这交通道路上重要的节点。它们纵横交贯，遍布全身，将人体内外、脏腑、肢节连成一个有机的整体。

According to TCM, there is a close connection between specific parts of the human body which is realized through specific meridians or collaterals. The connection was between points on the body surface and between a point the body surface and an internal organ. The meridian system is like a traffic system, consisting of main roads, auxiliary roads, and branches. Among them, the meridians are dominant, including twelve meridians and eight extra meridians; the collaterals are auxiliary, including the fifteen collaterals, twelve meridian sinews, and twelve cutaneous regions, etc.; the tertiary collaterals and superficial collaterals are branches. Each acupoint is an important intersection of roads or branches on the traffic system. They run throughout the body vertically and horizontally, connecting the inside and outside of the body, organs, limbs, joints, etc. into an organic whole.

在健康状态下,人体气血通过经络输送到各个脏腑、五官四肢,发挥其营养机体、抵御外邪的作用。同时,人体各系统通过经络的联系、沟通作用,构成一个彼此联系、配合的整体。在疾病状态下,经络又成为病邪传播和反映病变的途径,并能反映出疾病的病变部位。比如我们在头痛发作时,可以根据经脉在头面的分布和疼痛部位来判断病变的脏腑。如前额疼痛多与阳明经有关,头两侧疼痛多属少阳经病变,后脑及颈部疼痛多与太阳经有关。

根据经络具有传导信息、调节气血的功能,我们可以通过针刺、艾灸、推拿等治疗方法,对人体穴位给予适当的刺激,从而激发经络的调节功能来防治疾病。

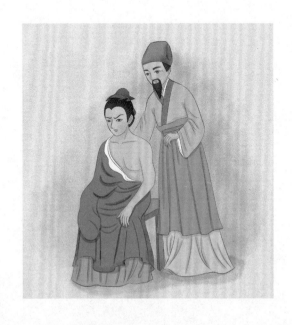

When a person is healthy, the qi and blood, transported through the meridians and collaterals to each internal organ, the head and limbs, and other parts of the body, fulfil the function of nourishing the body and resisting disease-causing factors. Meanwhile, the various systems of the body form a interrelated whole through the connection of the meridians. When a person is ill, the meridians and collaterals become the conduit through which a pathogenic factor is transmitted or a pathogenic change or the site of a disease is reflected. For example, when we have a headache, we can judge what internal organ is diseased based on the distribution of meridians in the head and the site of pain. In general, the pain in the forehead is related to the yangming channel, the pain at the temples is related to the shaoyang channel, and the pain in the back of the head and neck is related to the taiyang channel.

As the meridians have the function of transmitting information and regulating the circulation of qi and blood, we can give appropriate stimulation to the acupoints on the body surface through acupuncture, moxibustion, *tuina* (massage) and other treatments, so as to activate the regulating function of the meridians to prevent and cure diseases.

第三单元 中药与方剂

中药是以中国传统医药理论指导采集、炮制、制剂,说明作用机理,指导临床应用的药物。由于中药以植物药居多,故有"诸药以草为本"的说法。中药学是中医学的重要组成部分。中药是中医治病的主要手段,方剂就是治病的药方。中国古代很早已使用单味药物治疗疾病。经过长期的医疗实践,又学会将几种药物配合起来,经过煎煮制成汤液,即是最早的方剂。因此学习中药和方剂知识,对了解中药知识十分重要。

Unit Ⅲ Chinese Herbal Medicines & Formulas

There are a great variety of Chinese medicines, including plants, animal parts and minerals, which are collected, processed, prepared, and clinically applied under the guidance of Chinese traditional medicine theories. The majority of the materials are herbal, so Chinese medicinals are usually called Chinese herbal medicines. Chinese pharmacology, the scientific study of the source, collection, preparation, properties and efficacy of Chinese medicinal substances, is an essential part of Traditional Chinese Medicine (TCM). Medicinals, one of the major means of treating diseases, are usually compatibly put together to make formulas, based on the diagnosis of diseases and the properties and dosages of medicinals. It was recorded that single-medicinal formulas were used to treat diseases in ancient China. After a long period of practice, medicinals were compatibly combined and boiled for decoction (medicated liquid). The medicinals used in a combined manner for better efficacy were the earliest form of formulas. So, it is very important to acquire the knowledge of Chinese medicinal materials and formulas.

　　本单元将给大家讲述中药的起源、四气五味、加工、炮制、煎煮、服用方法，介绍道地药材的基本概念，讲述经典名方、国宝名药。我们还将带领大家一起认识"药食同源"的中国食疗文化。

This unit gives a brief introduction to the origins, four properties and five flavors of Chinese herbal medicines, and to the methods of processing medicinals, preparing decoction and taking decoction, as well as to the basic concepts of authentic medicinal materials, the knowledge of classical formulas and precious medicinals. It will also introduce you to the long-standing practice of dietary therapies in Chinese culture, where foods are regarded as being able to prevent and treat diseases as effectively as common medicinal herbs.

第十一章　中药的起源与传承

中药起源很早,可以追溯到原始社会,有数千年的悠久历史,是中国人民在长期的生产劳动、生活实践与医疗实践中,与疾病做斗争的过程中探索出来的。

远古时期,中药知识只能依靠师承口授,后来有了文字,便逐渐记录下来,出现了医药书籍。由于中药中草药类占大多数,所以记载药物的书籍便称为"本草"。现知最早的本草著作称为《神农本草经》,著者不详,根据其中记载的地名推测,可能是东汉医家修订前人著作而成。

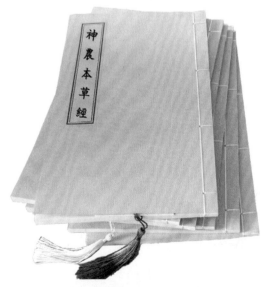

《神农本草经》古籍
An Ancient Version of the *Shennong Bencao Jing*
(*Shennong's Herbal*)

Chapter 11 Origins & Inheritance of Chinese Herbal Medicines

The origin of Chinese medicinals that have been studied and used for thousands of years can be traced back to the primitive society, when knowledge of all medicinal materials was acquired from the experience by Chinese people in their long struggle against diseases.

In ancient times, medicinal expertise could be passed down only by word of mouth, and later, more could be recorded by written words, which finally led to the appearance of books on medicals. A book on Chinese medicinals was normally called a "herbal" or a "book on herb medicine", for herbs accounted for the majority of all medicinal materials. The earliest existing book on herbal medicine is the *Shennong Bencao Jing* (*Shennong's Herbal*), with its authorship still unknown. According to the names of place mentioned in the book, it could be inferred that the book might be a revised version of the manuscript written by a great physician in the Eastern Han dynasty (25-220 AD).

《神农本草经》全书共三卷,收载药物包括动物、植物、矿物三类,共365种,每种药物词条下载有性味、功能与主治。另有序例简要地记述了用药的基本理论,如有毒无毒、四气五味、配伍法度、服药方法及丸、散、膏、酒等剂型,可说是汉代以前中医药物知识的总结,并为以后的药学发展奠定了基础。

到了南北朝,梁代陶弘景将《神农本草经》整理补充,著成《本草经集注》一书,其中增加了《名医别录》所用药物365种。

The *Shennong Bencao Jing* consists of three volumes, listing 365 medicinals from animals, plants and minerals, each having detailed descriptions of its properties, flavors, functions, and indications. In addition, basic applications of medicinals are briefly presented in its preface, in terms of toxicity or non-toxicity, four properties and five flavors, compatibility or incompatibility, methods of administration, and dosage forms such as pills, powders, ointments, medicated wine, etc. The book can be said to have been a summary of the knowledge of medicinals before the Han dynasty and to have laid a good foundation for the future development of pharmacology.

Tao Hongjing (456-536 AD), a great physician in the Liang of the Southern dynasties, revised and supplied notes to the *Shennong Bencao Jing* and wrote the *Bencao Jing Jizhu* (*Annotations to Shennong's Herbal*), which added 365 medicinals used by the famous doctors in the *Mingyi Bielu* (*Miscellaneous Records of Famous Physicians*).

到了唐代,由于生产力的发展以及对外交流日益频繁,外国药物陆续输入,药物品种日渐增加。为了适应形势需要,政府指派李绩等人主持增修本草经,称为《唐本草》。后来苏敬等重加修正,增药114种,于显庆四年(公元659年)颁行,称为《新修本草》或《唐新本草》,此书是中国也是世界上最早的一部药典。这部本草载药850种,并附有药物图谱,开创了中国本草著作图文对照的先例,不但对中国药物学的发展有很大影响,而且不久即流传国外,对世界医药的发展做出了重要贡献。

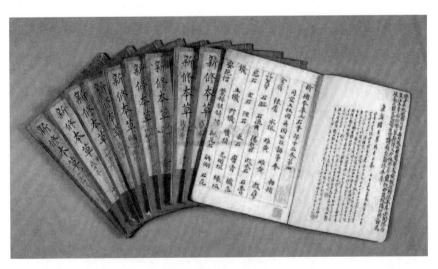

《新修本草》古籍
Xin Xiu Bencao (Newly-Revised Herbal)

In the Tang dynasty, the development of productive forces and increasing communications with foreign countries facilitated more medicinals being imported and increasing variety of medicinals being offered. In order to meet the needs of the new situation, Li Ji (594-669 AD), a famous general and good doctor, together with other famous doctors, was officially appointed to for the revisions of Tao Hongjing's book, and the new version was named the *Tang Bencao* (*Tang-Dynasty Herbal*). Later, Su Jing (599-674 AD), together with other herbalists, made corrections to it, and 114 medicinals were added. The revised book, published in 659 AD, was named the *Xin Xiu Bencao* (*Newly-Revised Herbal*) or *Tang Xin Bencao* (*Tang Xiu Bencao* (*New Tang-Dynasty Herbal*), which has been regarded as the earliest collection of medicinal materials in China and even in the world. It lists 850 materials with illustrations, setting an example for future illustrated herbals in China. The herbal not only had a great impact on the development of Chinese pharmacology, but was also soon spread abroad, making an important contribution to the development of world medicine.

　　明代伟大的医药学家李时珍结合自身经验和调查研究,穷搜博采,参考历代有关书籍资料八百余种,历时三十年,三次易稿而成《本草纲目》。

　　《本草纲目》全书约190万字,收录诸家本草所收药物1518种,在此基础上增收药物374种,辑录古代药学家和民间单方11096则,此外,还附药物形态图1100余幅。不仅详细描述了各种药物的形态、采集、炮制方法,还记录了药物的性味、归经、功效、主治等,使得药物学知识更加直观易懂,被誉为"东方药物学百科全书"。

　　《本草纲目》的特点在于其分类体系的科学性和系统性。李时珍根据药物的自然属性和医疗用途,将药物分为水部、火部、土部、金石部、草部、谷部、菜部、果部、木部、服器部、虫部、鳞部、介部、禽部、兽部、人部等16部,每部下又分若干类。这种分类方法在当时是非常先进的,对后世的药物学研究产生了深远影响。

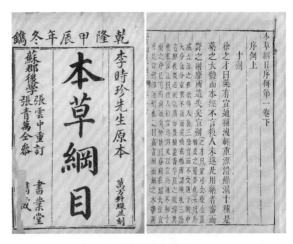

《本草纲目》古籍
An Ancient Version of the *Bencao Gangmu*
(*A Compendium of Materia Medica*)

Li Shizhen, a great pharmacist in the Ming dynasty, combined his own experience with investigation and research, read extensively, referenced more than 800 types of books and materials from previous dynasties, and spent 30 years completing the third and final draft of the *Bencao Gangmu* (*A Compendium of Materia Medica*) .

The *Bencao Gangmu* is approximately 1.9 million words and lists 1,518 types of medicinal substances recorded in various pharmacopeias. Additionally, it adds 374 substances, compiling a list of 11,096 recipes from ancient pharmacologists and folk remedies. Moreover, it is also provides over 1,100 illustrations of materials. It not only provides detailed descriptions of the morphology, collection, and processing methods of various substances but also those of their properties, flavors, meridian entries, efficacy, and main indications. This makes its readers to acquire the knowledge about Chinese medicines more easily and vividly, earning it the title of an encyclopedia of eastern pharmacology.

The characteristic of the *Bencao Gangmu* lies in its scientific and systematic classification. Li Shizhen categorized substances into sixteen types based on their natural properties and medical functions: Water, Fire, Earth, Metals and Stones, Herbs, Cereals, Vegetables, Fruits, Woods, Clothing and Utensils, Insects, Scales, Shells, Birds, Beasts and Humans, with each type further divided into several subtypes. This classification was very advanced in his day and had a profound impact on the study of pharmacology for later generations.

这部著作吸收了历代本草著作的精华,尽可能地纠正了以前的错误,补充了不足,并有很多重要发现和突破,是到16世纪为止中国最系统、最完整、最科学的一部医药学著作,对中国乃至世界医学和自然科学的发展产生了深远的影响。它被翻译成多种语言,成为世界医学史上的重要文献。

浩瀚的本草古籍是中医药学丰厚的文献资源,其所承载的中医药知识为中医药的学习、研究、传承和创新发挥着重要作用。

This work absorbs the essence of pharmacopeial writings from previous dynasties, correcting previous errors as much as possible, supplementing deficiencies, and making many important discoveries and breakthroughs. It was the most systematic, comprehensive, and scientific medical work in China up to the 16th century, having a profound impact on the development of medicine and natural sciences in China and the world. It has been translated into many languages and become an important document in the history of world medicine.

The vast array of ancient herbal texts constitutes a rich resource for TCM, playing a vital role in the study, research, inheritance, and innovation of TCM knowledge.

第十二章　中药的药性理论

中药药性理论即研究中药的性质、性能及其运用规律的理论。中药药性理论是中药理论的核心,主要包括四气、五味、归经、升降沉浮、有毒无毒等。

四气,就是寒、热、温、凉四种不同的药性,又称四性。它反映了药物对人体阴阳盛衰、寒热变化的作用倾向,为药性理论重要组成部分,是说明药物作用的主要理论依据之一。能够减轻或消除热症的中药,一般属于寒性或凉性,比如黄连、葛根等。反之,能够减轻或消除寒症的中药,一般属于温性或热性,比如附子、肉桂等。另外,还有一种平性,典型的例子就是甘草,主要起调和药性的作用。

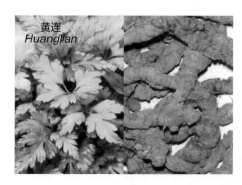
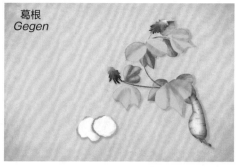

黄连
Huanglian

葛根
Gegen

寒凉性中药
Herbs with Cold and Cool Properties

Chapter 12 Properties of Chinese Herbal Medicines

The theories on properties of Chinese herbal medicines in general are mostly about their nature, properties, functions and applications. As the core of the theories, those on medicinal properties mainly deals with the four properties, five flavors, meridian entry, ascending or descending, toxicity or non-toxicity, etc.

The four properties refers to the four attributes of being cold, hot, warm and cool, which reflect the functional tendency of medicinal materials towards recovering a balance between yin and yang and causing the change of cold and heat in the human body. As an essential part of the theory of medicinal properties, the concepts in this respect provide one of the main theoretical bases for explaining the effects of medicinals. Medicinal herbs that can alleviate or eliminate heat symptoms are generally cold or cool in nature, such as *huanglian* (golden thread) and *gegen* (kudzu vine root). On the contrary, ones that can alleviate or eliminate cold symptoms are generally warm or hot, such as *fuzi* (prepared common monkshood root), *rougui* (cassia bark), and so on. In addition, there is an attribute of being neutral. A typical example is *gancao* (licorice root), which mainly plays the role of harmonizing the actions of ingredients of a formula.

　　五味,是指药物有酸、苦、甘、辛、咸五种不同的味道,相应地具有不同的治疗作用。有些还具有涩味或者淡味,因而实际上不止五种。但是,五味是最基本的五种滋味,所以仍然称为五味。

　　辛:"能散,能行",即具有发散、行气行血的作用。

　　甘:"能补,能和,能缓",即具有补益、和中、调和药性和缓急止痛的作用。

　　酸:"能收,能涩",即具有收敛、固涩的作用。

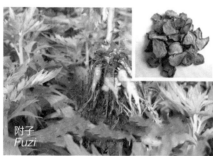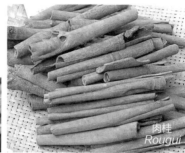

温热性中药
Herbs with Hot and Warm Properties

The five flavors refer to the sour, bitter, sweet, pungent and salty flavors of medicinal materials, which thus have separate therapeutic effects. Some are more astringent or milder, so there are actually more than five flavors. However, the five flavors are the most basic, which is why medicinal flavors are still limited to five.

Medicinals, which are pungent in nature, "disperse or mobilize", that is, they have the function of dispersing external pathogenic factors, and promoting the circulation of qi and blood.

Medicinals, sweet in nature, "tonify, harmonize, and moderate", that is, they have the functions of being tonic or nourishing, regulating the stomach, harmonizing medicinal properties if they are too powerful, and relieving pain.

Medicinals, sour in nature, "contract or control", namely they bear contracting or controlling effects, for example, checking sweating or arresting discharge.

苦：“能泄，能燥，能坚”，即具有清泄火热、泄降气逆、通泄大便、燥湿、坚阴的作用。

咸：“能下，能软”，即具有泻下通便、软坚散结的作用。

归经，是指药物对于机体某部分的选择性作用，即某药对某些脏腑经络有特殊的亲和作用，因而对这些部位的病变起着主要或特殊的治疗作用，药物的归经不同，其治疗作用也不同。

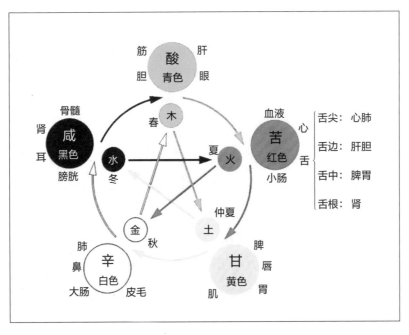

五行五色五味五季五脏六腑对应关系图

Medicinals, bitter in nature: "reduce, dry, or strengthen", that is, they have the function of reducing heat, reversing adverse motion of qi, purging stool, drying dampness, and strengthening yin, or quelling fire and preserving yin.

Medicinals, salty in nature: "lubricate the large intestine, or soften hard mass", that is, they have the function of purging stool and disintegrating masses.

The meridian entry refers to the selective action of a medicinal material on a particular part of the body, that is, a medicinal has a special affinity for a certain organ and/or meridians, thus playing a major or specific therapeutic role in relieving pathological factors in these body parts. The therapeutic effect of a medicinal depends on what meridian it enters.

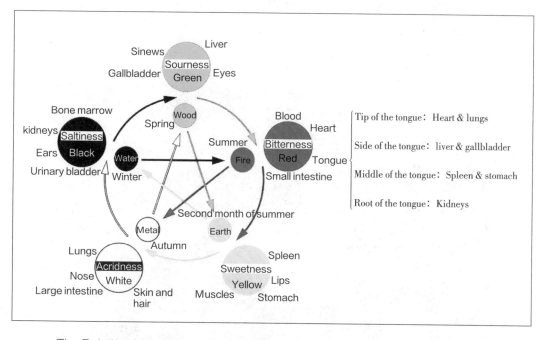

The Relationships Among the Five elements, Five Colours, Five Flavours, Five Seasons, Five Zang-organs and Six Fu-organs

第十三章　中药的炮制

　　中药必须经过炮制之后才能入药,是中医用药的特点之一。中药炮制是根据中医药理论,依照辨证施治用药的需要和药物自身性质,以及调剂、制剂的不同要求所采取的制药技术。2006年5月,中药炮制技术被列入第一批国家级非物质文化遗产名录传统医药类。

　　中药炮制是中医长期临床用药经验的总结。炮制工艺的确定以临床需求为依据,经炮制的中药在性味、功效、作用趋向、归经和毒副作用方面都会发生某些变化,从而最大限度地发挥疗效。因此,炮制工艺是否合理、方法是否恰当,直接影响到临床疗效。

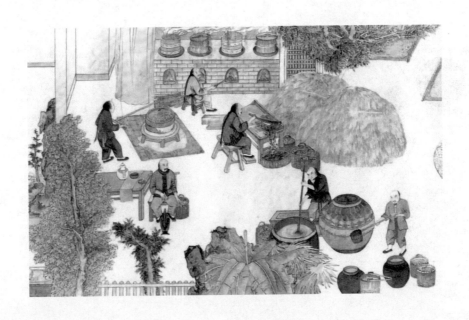

Chapter 13 Processing of Chinese Herbal Medicines

A Chinese medicinal material must be processed before it can be used for treatment, this being one of the characteristics of all medicinals. The processing is of a pharmaceutical technology based on the theory of Traditional Chinese Medicine (TCM), with a view to the needs of syndrome differentiation and treatment, the very nature of medicinals, and the different requirements of dispensing and preparing. In May 2006, the technique of Chinese medicine processing was included in the first batch of the National List of China Intangible Cultural Heritage under the category of traditional medicine.

Chinese herbal processing is the culmination of long-term clinical experience in TCM. The determination of processing techniques is based on clinical needs, and processed Chinese herbs undergo certain changes in properties, flavor, efficacy, action tendencies, meridian entry, and side effects, thereby maximizing their therapeutic effects. Consequently, whether the processing technique is reasonable and the method appropriate directly affects clinical efficacy.

传统的炮制方法主要有净制、切制、蒸、煮、炒、焙、炮、煅、浸、飞等,每种方法根据临床需求又采用不同的处理技术。如蒸,分为清蒸、酒浸蒸、药汁蒸;煮,分为盐水煮、甘草水煮、黑豆汁煮;炙,分为蜜炙、酥蜜炙、猪脂炙、药汁涂炙;浸,分为盐水浸、蜜水浸、米泔水浸、浆水浸、药汁浸、酒浸、醋浸等。以下摘录一些常见方法,供大家了解。

水飞:利用不同细度的药材粉末在水中的悬浮性不同而取得极细粉,并除去水溶性杂质的方法。

镑片:将经软化的药材用镑刀或镑片机镑成极薄片。

水研:指研粉时在研钵内加少量清水同研,研至符合规定时倾出,晾干。

武火:指大而猛的火。

Conventional processing methods mainly include purifying, cutting, steaming, boiling, stir-baking, baking, quick frying, calcining, soaking, grinding and so on, each method adopts different processing techniques according to clinical needs. For example, steaming is done with water, or wine, or a medicated juice. Boiling can be with salted water, with *gancao* (licorice root) juice, or with black bean juice. Stir-frying with liquid can be with honey, or crisp honey, or lard, or a medicated juice; soaking is with salted water, honey water, water of washing rice, *jiangshui* (fermented acid solution), a medicated juice, wine, or vinegar and so on. Here are some common methods.

Water-flying: obtain very fine powder in water and remove water-soluble impurities according to different suspension force of powder in various sizes.

Slicing: cut a softened medicinal material into very small thin slices with a special knife or cutting machine.

Water grinding: grind a medicinal together with a small amount of water in the mortar. After the grinding has reached the required standard, pour the ground medicinal out and dry it naturally.

Strong fire: big and fierce fire.

文火：指小而缓的火。用文火加热的锅，温度约为110～130℃。

酒蒸制：将净药材或切制品，加入定量的黄酒，拌匀。至酒渗入药材组织内部，然后置锅内蒸至符合规定。取出，干燥或做进一步加工。

姜蒸制：取规定量的鲜生姜，洗净，压榨取汁，与药材或切片拌匀，闷至姜汁渗入药材组织内部，置锅中用武火加热蒸至符合规定时取出，干燥。

醋炖制：将经预处理的净药材或切片与定量的米醋拌匀，闷至醋液渗入药材组织内部，然后将药材和未吸收完的醋液一并装入炖罐内，加盖。隔水炖至符合规定时取出，干燥或进一步加工。

Slow fire: small and gentle fire. The temperature of the pot heated by slow fire is about 110-130 degrees Celsius.

Steaming with wine: add a specified amount of yellow rice wine to cleaned or sliced material and mix them well. After the material be infiltrated by the wine, steam it in a pan until it has met the requirements. Then take it out to dry or further process it.

Steaming with ginger: mix the juice, which is squeezed from a specified amount of fresh ginger, with the medicinal material thoroughly, cover the material tightly until the ginger juice infiltrates the medicinal, and steam it in a pan with strong fire until it has met the requirements. Then take it out and dry it.

Stewing with vinegar: mix cleaned medicinal material with a certain amount of rice vinegar thoroughly until the vinegar infiltrates into the medicinal, put the medicinal and the vinegar left into a stewing pot, and cover the pot with a lid. And then put the pot into the pan with water in it and stew until the medicinal has met the requirements. Then take it out to dry or further process it.

炒黄:又称"炒香"。指用文火或武火将药材或生片炒至表面呈微黄色或深黄色(但不焦),此时可闻到药材固有的香气。

炒焦:指用文武火将药材或生片炒至表面焦褐色,内部颜色加深。方法为:先用武火将铁锅加热至现热焰,加入药材不断翻炒,并改用文武火加热,炒至符合规定时取出摊凉。

炒炭:用武火将药材或生片炒至表面焦黑色(炭化),内部呈焦褐色。方法为:先将炒锅用武火加热至投入少量药材即冒白烟时,将药物全部倒入锅内,翻炒至药材炭化即喷洒清水熄灭,取出放凉晒干。

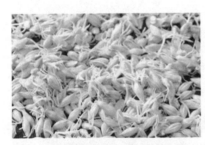

麦芽
Maiya (geminated barley)

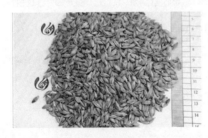

炒麦芽
Chaomaiya (parched geminated barley)

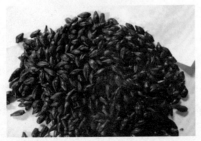

焦麦芽
Jiaomaiya (scorched geminated barley)

Stir-baking to yellow: also known as stir-baking to make it fragrant. Stir-bake medicinal materials with slow or strong fire until its surface has got yellowish or dark yellow (but not burnt), at which time the fragrance of the medicinal can be smelled.

Stir-baking to brown: stir-bake a medicinal material with a strong and then slow fire until its surface is brown or burnt and the internal color darkened. The method comprises the following steps: heat an iron pan with a strong fire until the bottom of the pan is burning hot, put the medicinal in, stir it nonstop, then heat it with a slow fire, and take out and cool the medicinal after it has met the requirements.

Stir-baking to get it carbonized: stir-bake a medicinal material with a strong fire until its surface is scorched or charred and the interior color brown but its medicinal property is not destroyed. The method is as follows: heat a frying pan with a strong fire until white smoke appears immediately after a small amount of medicinal material is added in, put all the medicinal material into the frying pan, and spray clear water to extinguish the smoke after the medicinal has got scorched. Then take it out to get cool and dry.

土炒：以土为辅料的一种伴炒法。方法为：将灶心土或陈土或赤石脂粉碎成细粉，置锅内，用武火加热翻炒至轻松流动状时加入药材，改用文火加热，翻炒至药材表面呈土色，透出药材固有香气时取出，筛去土，摊凉即可。

蜜制：系以蜂蜜为辅料的炙法的一种。方法为：取定量的炼蜜，加适量的开水稀释，将净药材或切制品与蜜水拌匀，闷至蜜水透入药材组织内部，置锅内，用文火加热翻炒至不黏手或规定程度。取出，放凉，密封保存。

Stir-baking with earth: a method of stir-baking with the auxiliary material earth. The method comprises the following steps: crush burned core earth from a stove or old wall earth or red halloysite into fine powder, put the powder into a pot, heat and stir-bake it with a strong fire until it flows like liquid, add the medicinal in, heat it with a slow fire and stir-bake it until its surface looks like earth in color and its fragrance emits and be smelled. Then take it out and let it cool for storage or future use.

Processing with honey: a metod of frying medicinal material with honey as the adjuvant. The method comprises the following steps: add a small amount of refined honey to boiled water, mix the cleaned material with the honey water thoroughly until it is infiltrated by the water, place the mixture in a pot, and heat and stir-fry the material with a slow fire until it is not sticky or meets the specified requirements. Then take the medicinal out, let it cool, and seal and store it.

第十四章　中药的配伍

我们所患的各种疾病都是由多种病邪及病因所致,单用一种中药不可能达到全面治愈疾病的目的,因此,必须根据疾病的病因,有选择地将多种药物配合同用。此外,各种中药都有其性味和归经,它们的药效、作用也不相一致。有的药物能补气,有的能活血,有的能理气,有的能解表,还有的药物能散寒等。而且药与药之间会发生某些相互作用,如有的能增强或降低原有药效,有的则能产生或增强毒副反应。因此,在使用中药时,必须有所选择。前人把中药之间的配伍关系总结为七个方面,称为药物的"七情"。现介绍如下。

相须:即性能功效相类似的药物配合应用,可以增强其原有疗效。如石膏与知母配合,能明显地增强清热泻火的治疗效果;大黄与芒硝配合,能明显地增强攻下泻热的治疗效果。

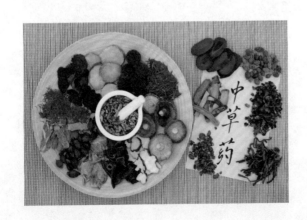

Chapter 14　Combinations of Chinese Herbal Medicines

Our diseases are usually caused by a variety of pathogens and causes, for which, in most cases, a single Chinese medicinal is unable to achieve the purpose of curing. Therefore, against the causes of a disease, two or more medicinals have to be selectively used in combination. What's more, all kinds of Chinese medicinals are different in nature, taste, entry, function and efficacy. For example, some materials can reinforce or regulate qi, some can improve blood circulation, some relieve an exterior symptom, and some dispel cold. Moreover, there are interactions between medicinals used in combination, and such interactions can enhance or reduce the original efficacy of medicinals, or even can bring about or enhance toxicity or side effects. Therefore, when using herbs, we have to be selective. Great physicians in Chinese history divided the combined application of medicinals in a formula into seven aspects, which are also called "seven principles of compatibility". Here are some main points.

Mutual accentuation, i. e. the combination of medicinals similar in function and efficacy, can enhance their original therapeutic properties. For example, a combined application of *shigao* (gypsum) and *zhimu* (rhizoma anemarrhenae) can significantly enhance the therapeutic effect of clearing heat and purging fire; while the combination of *dahuang* (rhubarb) and *mangxiao* (sodium sulfate) can significantly enhance the therapeutic effect of expelling heat by purgation.

相使:即在性能功效方面有某种共性的药物配合应用,而以一种药物为主,另一种药物为辅,能提高主药物的疗效。如补气利水的黄芪与利水健脾的茯苓配合时,茯苓能提高黄芪补气利水的治疗效果;清热泻火的黄芩与攻下泻热的大黄配合时,大黄能提高黄芩清热泻火的治疗效果。

相畏:即一种药物的毒性反应或副作用,能被另一种药物减轻或消除。如生半夏和生南星的毒性能被生姜减轻和消除,所以说生半夏和生南星畏生姜。

相杀:即一种药物能减轻或消除另一种药物的毒性或副作用。如生姜能减轻或消除生半夏和生南星的毒性或副作用,所以说生姜杀生半夏和生南星的毒。由此可知,相畏、相杀实际上是同一配伍关系的两种提法,是药物间相互对待而言的。

Mutual assistance, that is, the application of medicinals with common qualities in terms of property and effectiveness, with one as the main and other(s) as the supplement, can improve the therapeutic effect of the main medicinal. For example, when *huangqi* (milkvetch root) for reinforcing qi and promoting urine excretion is utilized together with *fuling* (Indian bread) for promoting urine excretion and invigorating the spleen, the latter can help improve the therapeutic effect of milkvetch root; when *huangqin* (baical skullcap root) for clearing heat and purging fire is used in combination with rhubarb for purging heat, the latter is able to improve the therapeutic effect of the former.

Mutual counteraction means that the toxic reaction or side effect of one medicinal can be reduced or eliminated by another. For example, the toxicity of *banxia* (pinellia tuber) and *tiannanxing* (jackinthepulpit tuber) is reduced or eliminated by *shengjiang* (fresh ginger), so the former ones cannot be used together with the latter.

Mutual suppression means that toxicity or adverse effects of one medicinal can be reduced or eliminated by another. For example, *shengjiang* can lessen or gets rid of the toxicity or side effects of *banxia* and *tiannanxing*, so *shengjiang* is used to suppress the toxicity of the above two. It can be seen from this that mutual counteraction and mutual suppression are actually two different expressions of the same combination, depending on which of the two used in combination is being concerned here.

119

相恶：即两种药物合用，一种药物与另一药物相作用而致原有功效降低，甚至丧失药效。如人参恶莱菔子，因莱菔子能削弱人参的补气作用。

相反：即两种药物合用，能产生毒性反应或副作用。如"十八反""十九畏"中的若干药物。

中药配伍的成果就是方剂，方指医方，剂指调剂，方剂就是治病的药方。方剂一般由君药、臣药、佐药、使药四部分组成。

"君臣佐使"的提法最早见于《素问》，在《素问·至真要大论》中有"主病之谓君，佐君之谓臣，应臣之谓使"的记载。历代医家对其含义各有解释。

Mutual antagonism, means that, when two medicinals are used together, one acts upon the other, resulting in a reduction or even loss of the latter's original efficacy. For example, *renshen* (ginseng) antagonizes the action of *laifuzi* (radish seed), for the latter weakens the role of the former in reinforcing the qi.

Incompatibility means that the combination of two medicinals produces toxic or side effects, such as the medicinals listed in the "eighteen incompatibilities" and "nineteen antagonisms".

A formula for an illness is the very fruit of combined applications of Chinese medicinals. In Traditional Chinese Medicine (TCM), a *fangji* (formula) for treating a disease originally has two senses: a prescription (a list of ingredients) and preparation (process of preparing something for medical purposes). Formulas are generally composed of four types of medicinals: a sovereign one, minister ones, assistant ones and courier ones.

The concepts of "sovereign, minister, assistant and courier" was first found in the *Suwen* (*Basic Questions*). In the 74th Chapter of the book, the *Comprehensive Discourse on the Essentials on the Most Reliable*, it is stated that, "The medicinal governing the disease is called the sovereign, those assisting the sovereign are called the ministers, and those responding to the ministers are called the couriers". Generations of physicians, however, had different interpretations of the concepts.

君药：即对处方的主病起主要治疗作用的药物。它体现了处方的主攻方向，其药力居方中之首，是组方中不可缺少的药物。

臣药：是辅助君药加强治疗主病的药物。

佐药：意义一是为佐助药，用于治疗次要兼证的药物；二是为佐制药，用以消除或减缓君药、臣药的毒性或烈性的药物；三是为反佐药，即根据病情需要，使用与君药药性相反而又能在治疗中起相成作用的药物。

使药：意义一是引经药，引方中诸药直达病所的药物；二是调和药，即调和诸药的作用，使其合力祛邪，如牛膝、甘草就经常作为使药入方。

The sovereign medicinal in a formula refers to the ingredient that serves to provide the principal curative action on the main syndrome in a patient. It reflects the prime target the formula is aimed at and its potency ranks first among all the ingredients in the formula, so it is indispensable.

A minister medicinal is an ingredient that assists the sovereign to strengthen the treatment of the main syndrome.

Assisting Medicine: The first meaning is as an auxiliary medicine, used to treat secondary concurrent conditions; The second is as a medicine to counteract, which is used to eliminate or reduce the toxicity or intensity of the sovereign and minister medicines; The third is as a medicine that opposes the nature of the sovereign medicine but can play a complementary role in treatment according to the needs of the condition.

The courier medicinal refers to an ingredient in a formula which directs the action of other ingredients to the affected meridian or the chief site of the disease or infection. It also refers to an ingredient that coordinates the action of other ingredients in a formula so that they can work towards eliminating pathogenic factors. For example, *niuxi* (twotoothed achyranthes root) and *gancao* (liquorice root) often serve as courier medicials in recipes.

　　例如：《伤寒论》的麻黄汤，由麻黄、桂枝、杏仁、甘草四味药组成，主治恶寒发热、头疼身痛、无汗而喘、舌苔薄白、脉浮紧等，属风寒表实证。方中麻黄辛温解表，宣肺平喘，针对主证为君药；桂枝辛温解表，通达营卫，助麻黄峻发其汗为臣药；杏仁肃肺降气，助麻黄以平喘为佐药；甘草调和麻黄、桂枝峻烈发汗之性为使药。由于"君臣佐使"为封建政体名称，现多改称"主辅佐使"或"主辅佐引"。

　　用方如用将，用药如用兵。方剂中每一味中药各司其职，各尽其能，就能达到"增效减毒"的目的，这就是中药配伍的意义。

For example, the *Mahuang Decoction* listed in the *Shang-han Lun* (*Treatise on Exogenous Febrile Diseases*) is composed of *mahuang* (ephedra), *guizhi* (cassia twig), *kuxingren* (bitter apricot seed), and *gancao*. The formula is mainly used to allevi-ate symptoms of a wind-cold exterior excess syndrome, such as aversion to cold, fever, headache, a general aching, absence of sweating, asthma, a thin white tongue coating, a floating and tight pulse, etc. In the formula, *mahuang*, serving as the sovereign medicinal against the main syndrome, is pungent and warm for relieving an exterior syndrome, ventilating the lung to relieve asthma; *guizhi*, serving as the minister medici-nal, is pungent and warm for relieving an exterior syndrome, activating the nutritive and defensive levels, assisting ephedra in sweating; *kuxingren*, serves as the assistant medicinal for purifying the lung and descending the adversely risen qi, and assists *mahuang* in relieving asthma; and *gancao*, serves as the courier medicinal for moderating the action of *mahuang* and *guizhi* in case they are too powerful. The terms "sovereign, minister, assistant and courier" are actually official titles of the feudal society, so now we instead use the terms of "princi-pal, associate, assistant, and envoy" or "chief, deputy, assis-tant and conductive".

Deciding on a formula is like choosing a general, and us-ing medicinals is like dispatching soldiers to a battle. This means every single medicinal in a formula performs its own functions and duties to achieve the final purpose of "maximiz-ing efficacy and minimizing toxicity", which is the significance of combined applications of Chinese medicinals.

第十五章　源远流长的"药食同源"

　　"民以食为天"。饮食不但是人类赖以生存的物质基础,而且也与人类的健康息息相关。古代医学家将中药的"四性""五味"理论运用到食物之中,认为每种食物也具有"四性""五味"。"药食同源"是说中药与食物是同时起源的。《黄帝内经》中就有食疗的理论,如"谷肉果菜,食养尽之,无使过之,伤其正也。"唐朝时期的《黄帝内经·太素》一书中写道:"空腹食之为食物,患者食之为药物。"都反映了"药食同源"的思想。那么,"药食同源"的食物有哪些呢? 根据国家卫生健康委发布的药食同源目录,目前共有110种既是食品又是中药。现摘录部分药物,供大家了解。

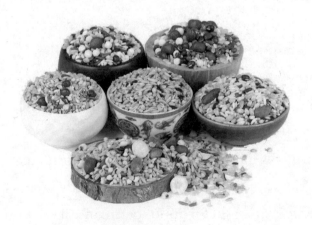

Chapter 15 The Long-Standing "Common Source of Medicine & Food"

"Food is the first necessity of the people". It is not only the basis for human survival, but also closely related to human health. Ancient physicians applied the principles of "four properties" and "five flavors" to food materials, believing that each food material also has its own property and flavor. This is what "food and medicine being of the common source" means in Traditional Chinese Medicine (TCM) or even in Chinese dietary culture. In the *Huangdi Neijing* (*Huangdi's Classic of Medicine*) there are very good discussions with regard to dietary therapy: "Then proper diets of grain, meat, fruit or vegetables are adopted to complete the cure. Do not permit these limits to be exceeded in case the proper is harmed. " In *Huangdi Neijing Taisu,* an earlier version of the *Huangdi Neijing*, published in the Tang dynasty, it is stated that "what is eaten in an empty stomach is food, while what is eaten by a patient is medicine", which has definitely reflected the idea of "medicine and food being the common source". So, what are the materials that are able to be regarded as both edible and medicinal? There are 110 kinds of medicinals on the official list issued by the National Health Commission of the People's Republic of China. Here are some of them.

　　聪耳(增强或改善听力)类食物:莲子、山药、荸荠、蒲菜、芥菜、蜂蜜。

　　明目(增强或改善视力)类食物:山药、枸杞、蒲菜、猪肝、羊肝、野鸭肉、青鱼、鲍鱼、螺蛳、蚌。

　　生发(促进头发生长)类食物:白芝麻、韭菜籽、核桃仁。

　　润发(使头发滋润、光泽)类食物:鲍鱼。

　　乌须发(使须发变黑)类食物:黑芝麻、核桃仁、大麦。

　　长胡须(有益于不生胡须的男性)类食物:鳖肉。

　　美容颜(使肌肤红润、光泽)类食物:枸杞子、樱桃、荔枝、黑芝麻、山药、松子、牛奶、荷蕊。

　　健齿(使牙齿坚固、洁白)类食物:花椒、蒲菜、莴笋。

　　轻身(消肥胖)类食物:菱角、大枣、榧子、龙眼、荷叶、燕麦、青粱米。

Materials that are helpful in improving hearing: *lianzi* (lotus seed), *shanyao* (common yam rhizome), *biqi* (water chestnut), *pucai* (cattail sprout), *jiecai* (leaf mustard), honey.

Materials that are helpful in protecting or improving eyesight: common yam rhizome, *gouqi* (barbary wolfberry fruit), cattail sprout, pork liver, sheep liver, wild duck meat, herring, abalone, river snail and mussel.

Materials that are helpful in promoting hair growth: white sesame seed, garlic chive seed, and walnut kernel.

Material that is helpful in making hair bushy and shiny: abalone.

Materials that are helpful in making hair blacker: black sesame seed, walnut kernel, and barley.

Material that is helpful in making a beardless man grow a beard: turtle meat.

Materials that are helpful in keeping the skin ruddy and shiny: barbary wolfberry fruit, cherry, lychee, black sesame seed, common yam rhizome, pine nut, milk, and *herui* (lotus pistil).

Materials that are helpful in keeping teeth firm and white: *huajiao* (pricklyash peel), cattail sprout, and lettuce.

Materials that are helpful in making fat people thinner and stronger: water caltrop, *dazao* (Chinese jujube or date), grand torreya seed, *longyan* (longan aril), lotus leaf, oat, and green sorghum rice.

肥人（改善瘦人体质，强身壮体）类食物：小麦、粳米、酸枣、葡萄、藕、山药、黑芝麻、牛肉。

增智（益智、健脑等）类食物：粳米、荞麦、核桃、葡萄、菠萝、荔枝、龙眼、大枣、百合、山药、茶、黑芝麻、黑木耳、乌贼鱼。

益志（增强志气）类食物：百合、山药。

安神（使精神安静、利睡眠等）类食物：莲子、酸枣、百合、梅子、荔枝、龙眼、山药、鹌鹑、牡蛎肉、黄花鱼。

增神（增强精神，减少疲倦）类食物：茶、荞麦、核桃。

强筋骨（强健体质，包括筋骨、肌肉以及体力）类食物：栗子、酸枣、黄鳝、食盐。

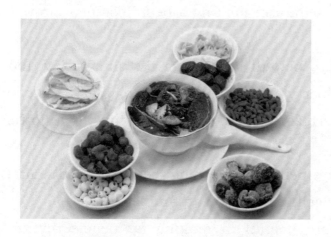

其实生活中常见的肥胖、青春痘、视力下降、失眠、上火等问题，都可以通过饮食调理来解决，具体的方法在后面的章节中还有介绍。

Materials that are helpful in rebuilding the constitution of very thin people and making them fatter and stronger: wheat, rice, *suanzao* (spine date), grape, lotus root, common yam rhizome, black sesame seed, and beef.

Materials that nourish the brain: rice, buckwheat, walnut kernel, grape, pineapple, lychee, longan aril, Chinese jujube or date, lily bulb, common yam rhizome, tea, black sesame seed, black fungus, cuttlefish.

Materials that are helpful in improving memory and will: lily bulb, common yam rhizome.

Materials that are helpful in resting the nerves, or inducing sleep: lotus seed, spine date, lily bulb, plum, lychee, longan aril, common yam rhizome, quail meat, oyster meat, and yellow croaker.

Materials that have restorative properties (which are helpful in lifting spirits and relieving tiredness): tea, buckwheat, walnut kernel.

Materials that are helpful in rebuilding the constitution, or making bones firmer and stronger, and making sinews, ligaments and muscles stronger and more powerful: chestnut, spine date, eel, salt.

In fact, common problems in daily life such as fatness or obesity, acne, weak or poor sight, sleeplessness, excessive internal heat that may cause a toothache or a sore throat, etc., can be solved through dietary adjustment, and the specific ways will be introduced in the following chapters.

第四单元　甘肃医药故事

　　甘肃地处黄土高原、青藏高原和内蒙古高原三大高原的交会地带，地貌复杂多样，光照充足，气候类型多样，出产了很多优质道地药材，比如岷县当归、陇西党参、文县纹党参、陇西黄芪、武都红芪、靖远枸杞、陇南大黄、民勤甘草等，还有柴胡、款冬花、秦艽、锁阳等。

Unit Ⅳ Stories Related to Medicine in Gansu

Gansu is located in the intersection zone of the Loess Plateau, the Qinghai-Xizang Plateau and the Inner Mongolia Plateau. Due to factors such as complex and diverse landforms, abundant sunlight, and various climate types, abundant authentic medicinal substances with high qualities are produced in Gansu, including *danggui* (Chinese angelica) in Minxian, *dangshen* (tangshen) in Longxi, *wendangshen* (striped tangshen) in Wenxian, *huangqi* (milkvetch root) in Longxi, *hongqi* (manyinflorescenced sweetvetch root) in Wudu, *gouqi* (barbary wolfberry fruit) in Jingyuan, *dahuang* (rhubarb root and rhizome) in Longnan, *gancao* (liquorice root) in Minqin, as well as *chaihu* (Chinese thorowax root), *kuandonghua* (common coltsfoot flower), *qinjiao* (largeleaf gentain root), and *suoyang* (songaria cynomorium herb), etc.

在孕育出诸多道地药材的同时，甘肃也为中华文明的延续和中医药学的诞生与发展书写了浓墨重彩的一笔，伏羲、岐伯、封衡、皇甫谧等甘肃历史人物为中医药学的发展做出了突出贡献。

本单元将给大家介绍甘肃道地药材和名老中医的故事。

While cultivating a multitude of authentic medicinal substances, Gansu has also contributed significantly to the continuation of the Chinese civilization and the birth and development of Traditional Chinese Medicine (TCM). Historical figures from Gansu such as Fuxi, Qi Bo, Feng Heng, and Huangfu Mi have made outstanding contributions to the development of TCM.

In this unit, some of the authentic medicinal substances in Gansu and stories of renowned TCM practitioners will be introduced to you.

第十六章　岷县当归香气浓

"曾子定应怜益母，曹公端解寄当归。从今洗面饶光泽，血气仍充旧带围。"宋代诗人朱翌的《有惠益母粉及当归者》道出了当归的功效。当归是常用的补血类中药，在中药方剂中比较常见，而在全国所产当归中，以甘肃岷县地区所产当归最好，称之为"岷归"，是中国国家地理标志产品。

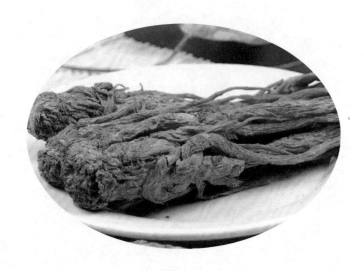

Chapter 16 Chinese *Danggui* Produced in Minxian

In the four-line poem *You Hui Yimu Fen Ji Danggui Zhe* (Benefiting from yimu motherwort powder) and *danggui* (Chinese angelica), the author clearly tells us the function and efficacy of *danggui*, "Zengzi (a great thinker in ancient China) was fond of *yimu*, and Cao Cao (an outstanding statesman in ancient China) understood the soldier's purpose of sending *danggui* to his mother; benefiting from these medical herbs, I feel my face glowing with health, and I can feel the blood and qi replenishing my old body." *Danggui* is a commonly used blood-enriching medical herb, and is frequently employed in Traditional Chinese Medicine (TCM) formulas. Of all *danggui* in the whole country, that produced in Minxian county and surrounding areas is the best. The variety is known as *Mingui* (abbreviation for Chinese angelica of Minxian) and is a geographical indication product of China.

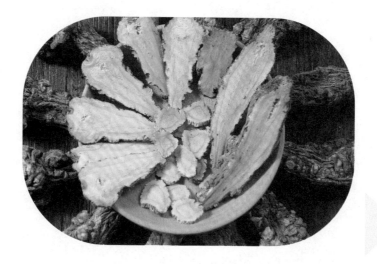

岷县当归的道地产区包括岷县、宕昌、临潭及卓尼等周边地区。《居延汉简》《武威汉代医简》和中国第一部中药专著《神农本草经》对"岷归"入药都有记载，至今已有2000多年的历史。据《梁书·宕昌国传》记载，公元505年，宕昌国王梁弥博来朝，献上甘草、当归。当时的宕昌国，即今甘肃的岷县、宕昌一带。可见，在1500多年前，"岷归"就已经作为贡品了。

Counties producing *danggui* in this region include Minxian, Tanchang, Lintan and Zhuoni, etc. *Mingui* has been used as a medical herb for more than 2,000 years, about which we can find some clues in the *Juyan Han Jian* (*Juyan Bamboo Slips from Han Dynasty*), *Wuwei Han Dai Yi Jian* (*Bamboo Slips from Han Dynasty Recording Traditional Chinese Medicine Unearthed in Wuwei*), and *Shennong Bencao Jing* (*Shennong's Classic of Materia Medica*) which is the first monograph on TCM. According to the *Liang Shu Tanchang Guo Zhuan* (*The Book of Liang, Records of the Kingdom of Tanchang*), in 505 A D, Liang Mibo, the ruler of Tanchang, came to court and offered *gancao* (liquorice root) and *danggui* to the emperor. The Tanchang realm at that time turned out to be the area of Minxian and Tanchang in present Gansu. Therefore, we have clear evidence that as early as 1,500 years ago, *Mingui* had already been used as tribute.

"岷归"属多年生草本,药用部位是当归干燥的根。"岷归"具有主根长、皮细质坚,且全株散发一种特异香气的特点。秋季采收,抖净泥沙,通风晾至半干,按大小扎成小把,架在烘架上用微火慢慢熏烤至八成干,表皮呈灰棕色或棕褐色后取下,让其自然干燥。使用前,水洗切片,干燥。另外入药还有当归炭和当归酒,当归炭是将当归片大火炒成浅黑色,洒水适量,取出晾凉。当归酒是将当归片用黄酒喷淋均匀,稍闷,用微火稍炒,取出放凉。

"岷归"是妇科要药,远销世界20多个国家或地区,在国内外有很高的声誉,有着"中华当归甲天下,岷县当归甲中华"的美誉。

Mingui is a perennial herb, and the part used as medicine is its dried roots. *Mingui* has the characteristics of a long tap-root and firm skin, the whole plant emitting a special aroma. To make *Mingui* medicinal, people would harvest its roots in autumn, clean off the mud and sand, air them until half-dry, and bunch them into small bundles as to their different sizes. The next step is to put the bundles on a drying rack, slowly smoke and roast them over a low fire until the roots are 80% dry, when the skins become grayish brown or brown. At last, let them dry out naturally. Before put to use, it would be washed, sliced, and then dried. *Danggui charcoal* and *danggui wine* are also used as medicine. The former is made by stir-frying *danggui slices* over high heat until they turn a light black color, then sprinkling them with a moderate amount of water and allowing them to cool. While *danggui wine* is made by evenly spraying *danggui slices* with yellow wine, slightly steaming, lightly stir-frying over low heat, and then allowing them to cool.

Mingui, exported to more than 20 countries or regions in the world, is an important gynecological medicine with a high reputation both domestically and internationally. It is said that "*Danggui* from China is the best in the world, and that from Minxian county is the best in China".

第十七章　党参三品齐争艳

党参是常用的补气类中药,因产于山西上党而得名,以质柔润、味甜者为佳。甘肃盛产党参,而且产量占到了全国的四分之三。在甘肃道地党参中,还细分了三个品种。

陇西白条党参

甘肃陇西白条党参是中国国家地理标志产品,在陇西县已有上千年的种植历史。陇西良好的种植条件造就了白条党参的优异品质,具有色白条直、皮紧、肉厚、味甘、嚼之无渣的特点,国内外用户赞誉不绝。白条党参有养血、健脾、补中、益气、降压、生津、抗癌的功效,常作为人参的代用品,俗称"小人参"。

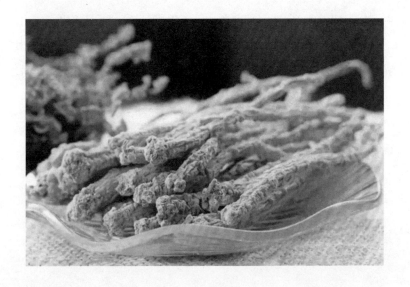

Chapter 17 Three Varieties of *Dangshen*

Dangshen (tangshen) is a commonly used medical herb for tonifying qi. It was named after a place named Shangdang (in Shanxi province) where *dangshen* was originally grown and is considered the best as it is soft and moist in texture and sweet in taste. Gansu is rich in *dangshen,* with its production accounting for three-quarters of the national output. Three varieties of authentic *dangshen* are produced in Gansu.

Longxi straight white dangshen

Longxi straight white dangshen from Gansu is a Chinese geographical indication product, with a cultivation history of over a thousand years in Longxi County. The excellent cultivation conditions in Longxi have resulted in the outstanding quality of *straight white dangshen.* It is characterized by its white color, straight rootstock, tight skin, thick flesh and sweet taste, with no dregs left when chewed, earning praise from users both domestically and internationally. *Straight white dangshen* is known for its blood-nourishing, spleen-strengthening, middle-tonifying, qi-boosting, blood pressure-lowering, thirst-quenching, and anticancer effects, due to which it is often used as a substitute for *renshen* (ginseng), thus commonly referred to as small ginseng.

渭源白条党参

甘肃省渭源县被誉为"中国党参之乡",所产党参称"渭源白条党参",是全国农产品地理标志。根呈长圆柱形,根长分枝少。顶端常有一膨大的根头(俗称狮子盘头)。外皮呈黄褐色或乳白色,上部有细密横纹,下部干燥后有纵纹。鲜根断裂处有白色胶状物溢出,干燥后呈黑色。横切面为微黄色菊花心形状,肉厚,体质坚实,气味特殊,嚼起来甘甜无渣。

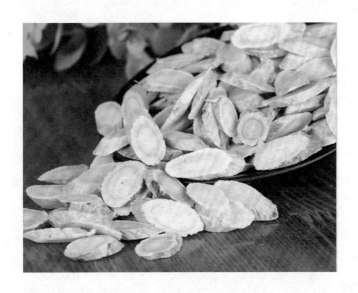

文县纹党参

纹党参是党参的一种,因其根表皮皱且密布横状环纹而得名。纹党参产区分布于甘肃陇南、陕西西南及四川西北部,因其主产于甘肃文县,又称"文党"。

Weiyuan straight white dangshen

Weiyuan County in Gansu is known as the hometown of *dangshen* in China, and *dangshen* produced there is called *Weiyuan straight white dangshen*, which is a national geographical indication of agricultural products. It is characterized by a long cylindrical root and few branches. Normally, it has a swollen root tip, with some tuberous stem scars. The skin is yellow-brown or milky white, with fine horizontal lines in the upper part, and longitudinal lines in the lower part when it becomes dry. A white gelatinous substance would overflow from a broken part of a fresh root, which turns black after drying, and the cross section displays a light-yellow chrysanthemum-like pattern. This variety also features thick flesh, solid texture, distinct smell, sweet taste and no residue when chewed.

Wenxian striped dangshen

There is another kind of *dangshen* called *striped dangshen*, which is named for its wrinkled root skin and horizontal ring-like patterns. It is mainly distributed in Longnan, Gansu, southwestern Shanxi, and northwestern Sichuan in China. As it is primarily produced in Wenxian county, Gansu, it is also known as *Wendang* (abbreviation for *Wenxian dangshen* in Chinese).

文县纹党参是甘肃四大名药之一,是中国国家地理标志产品。具有狮子盘头菊花心,外松内紧体柔韧,身长粗壮肉质厚,味清甜润嚼无渣,有细密横纹,通达根体过半等特征。《本草正义》记载,纹党参性能与人参相去不远,是党参中的上品,其有效药用成分含量居各类党参之首。因此,纹党参除有补中益气、健脾强身作用外,还对脾胃虚弱、血气亏损、体倦无力、贫血、白血病、妇女血崩、产后诸病有显著的疗效。纹党曾在中国各种党参评比中名列第一,荣获对外出口商品荣誉证书,远销世界130多个国家和地区,为甘肃大宗出口中药材,驰名中外。

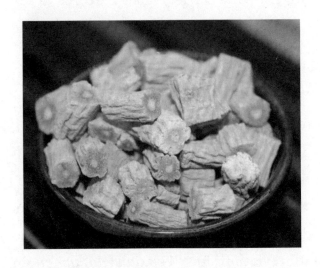

Wenxian striped dangshen is one of the four famous medicinal herbs in Gansu, and is a Chinese geographical indication product. It has characteristics such as a lion-shaped flower head with a chrysanthemum heart, soft and flexible outer layer but firm inner core, long and thick body with thick flesh that can be chewed without residue left, fine horizontal lines and long roots that are more than half of its body. It is recorded in the *Bencao Zhengyi* (*Expounding on the Classical Texts of Materia Medica*) that the efficacy of *striped dangshen* is very close to that of renshen, making it the top-grade *dangshen* with the content of its effective medicinal ingredients ranks first among all varieties. In addition to tonifying the middle and benefiting qi, invigorating the spleen, and strengthening the body, it also has remarkable therapeutic effects on conditions such as weakness in spleen and stomach, deficiency of blood and qi, fatigue, anemia, leukemia, women's excessive menstrual bleeding, and postpartum ailments. *Striped dangshen* once ranked first in various evaluations of *dangshen* in China and was awarded a certificate of honor of export commodities. It has been exported to over 130 countries and regions and has become a well-known Chinese herbal medicine both domestically and internationally.

第十八章 千古医宗话岐伯

岐伯是中国传说中远古时代最著名的医生，生卒年月不详。岐伯之名始见于《史记》，《汉书·艺文志·方技》在列数古代著名医家时记载道："太古有岐伯、俞拊，中世有扁鹊、秦和。"可见，岐伯是与黄帝同时代的人物。清代乾隆年间的《庆阳县志·人物》记载："岐伯，北地人，生而精明，精医术脉理，黄帝以师事之，著《内经》行于世，为医书之祖。"

Chapter 18 Qi Bo—An Outstanding Physician
in Ancient China

Qi Bo is the most famous ancient physician in Chinese legends, with his exact date of birth and death unknown. The name Qi Bo first appeared in the *Shi Ji* (*The Historical Records*). In the part of the *Han Shu Yi Wen Zhi Fang Ji* (*The Book of Han, Arts and Literature Category, Skills and Techniques*), which lists famous ancient physicians and mentions, "In ancient times there were Qi Bo and Yu Fu, in the mediaeval times there were Bianque and Qin He." It can be seen that Qi Bo lived in the same period as Huangdi. It was recorded in the *Qingyang Xian Zhi Renwu* (*Qingyang County Records, People*) from the Qianlong period in the Qing dynasty, "Qi Bo, a person from the northern region, was born intelligent, proficient in medical skills and pulse diagnosis. Huangdi studied under him, and wrote the *Huangdi Neijing* (*Huangdi's Classic of Medicine*), which spread throughout the world and became the cornerstone of Traditional Chinese Medicine.

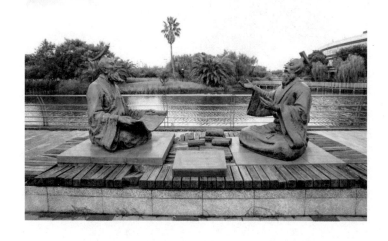

　　《黄帝内经》既是先秦医学思想与临床经验的一次总结，也是中国现存最早、最完备的中医学奠基之作，其主要内容是以黄帝、岐伯问答的体裁论医，并涉及天文、历法、气象、地理、生物、农艺、哲学、音乐等方面的知识。作为中医药学的第一部经典，它构建了中医药学的理论体系和基本框架，全面系统地介绍了养生保健知识，既是医家临证之书，更是古代的百科全书与中华传统文化的瑰宝。因此《黄帝内经》被尊称为"医家之宗"。从此，中医药学又称为"岐黄之术"。

　　岐伯知识渊博，在《黄帝内经》中，他精辟地回答了黄帝提出的1000多个问题，故"黄帝以师事之"。他明察哲理，通过分析诊断的疾病，阐述治国为政的道理。

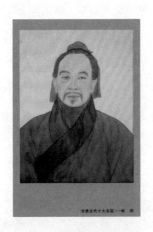

岐伯画像
Portrait of Qibo

The *Huangdi Neijing* is not only a summary of the medical thoughts and clinical experiences from the pre-Qin period, but also the earliest and most complete groundbreaking work of Traditional Chinese Medicine (TCM). It records the dialogues between Huangdi and Qi Bo, which are mainly around medical theories and involve knowledge in astronomy, calendar system, meteorology, geography, biology, agriculture, philosophy, music, etc. As the first classic in TCM, it established a theoretical system and basic framework for the discipline, and comprehensively and systematically introduced a knowledge of health preservation. It serves not only as a reference for medical practitioners but also as an encyclopedia of ancient times and a treasure of Chinese traditional culture. Therefore, the *Huangdi Neijing* has been revered as the bible of medical practitioners. And since then, TCM has been called Qi-Huang's medicine in China.

Qi Bo was knowledgeable, in the *Huangdi Neijing*, he provided insightful answers to over 1,000 questions posed by the Huangdi, therefore, he was regarded as a teacher by Huangdi. Qi Bo also had profound philosophical insights. By analyzing and diagnosing diseases, he elaborated on the principles of governing a country.

岐伯是中医学的奠基者,著述颇丰。他除以著《黄帝内经》行于世之外,据有关史志书目记载,岐伯的其他著作还有10种,全都已丢失,仅存书目,因此只能从书名知道这些著作与岐伯有关,内容主要是针灸,还有按摩、藏象等。

岐伯受到历代人民的尊崇,修祠建庙,以作纪念。2003年,庆阳市庆城县在周祖陵森林公园东山复建岐伯庙,每年三月初五的岐伯庙会,就是为了纪念出生在这块厚土上的远古圣贤岐伯而举行的。

Qi Bo was the founder of TCM and had a rich literary legacy. Legend has it that in addition to the widely known *Huangdi Neijing*, whose accomplishment was attributed to him, Qi Bo authored 10 other works, but all of which were lost and only their titles exist in bibliographic records. Therefore, we can only infer from those titles that they were related to Qi Bo and mainly focused on acupuncture, as well as massage, pulse diagnosis, and other topics.

Qi Bo has been highly revered by people from generation to generation, and shrines and temples in his honor have been built. In 2003, people in Qingcheng county, Qingyang city, reconstructed the Qi Bo Temple on the eastern hill of the Zhouzuling Forest Park. The annual Qi Bo Temple Fair held on the fifth day of the third lunar month is dedicated to worshipping and commemorating this ancient sage, who was born on this piece of land.

第十九章　针灸鼻祖皇甫谧

　　皇甫谧,字士安,自号玄晏先生,是中国历史上著名的学者,在医学、文学、史学诸方面都颇有建树。

Chapter 19 Huangfu Mi—Originator of Acupuncture and Moxibustion

Huangfu Mi, style-named Shi'an and self-titled as Sir Xu-anyan, was a renowned scholar in Chinese history, who made significant achievements in the fields of medicine, literature, and historiography.

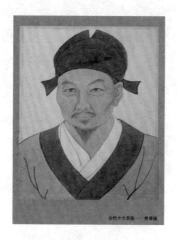

皇甫谧画像
Portrait of Huangfu Mi

皇甫谧六七岁时,由叔母任氏抚养,不好好读书,整天和同龄孩子游玩度日,无所作为,但与同辈交往很讲义气,对长辈很孝顺,常带瓜果一类食物回家给长辈吃。有一天,他又带回瓜果孝敬叔母,任氏让他坐在身边,痛心地教诲道,《孝经》记载孔子曰:"孝子之事亲也,居则致其敬,养则致其乐,病则致其忧,丧则致其哀,祭则致其严。五者备矣,然后能事亲。五者备矣,然后能事亲。事亲者,居上不骄,为下不乱,在丑不争。三者不除,虽日用三牲之养,犹为不孝也。"接着开导他说:"先前孟子的母亲为了孟子学好,三次搬家;曾子用杀猪的办法教子。我虽然比不上他们,但也够苦口婆心的了。你怎么一句也听不进去?你什么时候才能知道用功学习呢?"皇甫谧听了叔母的教诲和自责,难过得掉下了眼泪,跪泣叩首,表示从此痛改前非,发奋读书供养二老。

When Huangfu Mi was about six or seven years old, he was fostered by his aunt Ren. Instead of studying hard, he spent his days hanging around with children of the same age, doing nothing. Despite his underachievement, he was loyal to his peers and respectful to the elders, so he often brought home the food he got from others to share with elder members of the family. One day, when he took home some melons and fruits to give his aunt again, she, in distress, asked him to sit by her side and said, It is recorded in the *Xiao Jing* (*Classic of Filial Piety*) that Confucius once said, "The duties of a filial son to his parents are as follows: while at home, he should behave with the utmost respect; when taking care of his parents, he should do everything merrily; when they are ill, he should show the deepest concern; when mourning for their death, he should exhibit the sincerest grief; when sacrificing, he should display the utmost reverence. Only when he is qualified in these five aspects, can he really serve his parents. To serve the parents, one should also avoid being arrogant when in a high position, causing trouble when in a lower position, and engaging in fights among vulgar crowds. If one does not refrain from the three evils of arrogance, chaos, and fight, even if he diligently provides his parents with the choicest meats and the finest wines, he is still considered unfilial." She then reminded him of the efforts made by Mencius's mother, who moved their home three times for his education, and how Zengzi used a pig-killing incident to teach his son. She expressed her own efforts and pleaded with him to understand the importance of studying diligently. Touched by his aunt's words and feeling remorseful, Huangfu Mi tearfully knelt down, promising to mend his ways and study hard to support his elderly aunt and uncle.

　　他说到做到，很快拜有学问的席坦为师，努力学习，这样日复一日、年复一年，学业大有长进，品德也为乡人所敬仰。约在42岁，皇甫谧身患风痹病，半身麻木，疼痛不已；随后右足萎缩，行动不便；接着他又不幸患耳聋病，与人交谈困难。他便决心学医，很多人劝他做官，他写了《释劝论》表明心迹，立志兼学医术。

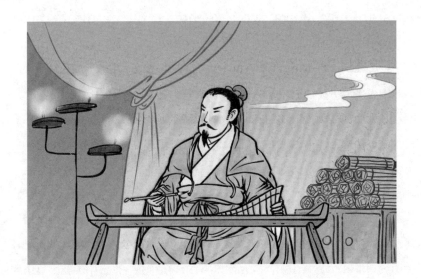

Huangfu Mi lived up to his words. He soon took Xitan, a knowledgeable man, as his teacher and studied hard. Day after day, year after year, he made great progress in his studies, and earned respect from his fellow villagers for his moral character. Around the age of 42, Huangfu Mi unfortunately developed moving impediment, leaving him half-body numbed and in constant pain. His right foot atrophied, making movement difficult. Subsequently, he suffered from deafness, making it difficult to talk with others. Despite many advising him to pursue an official career, he was determined to study medicine. To express his intentions and aspirations, he wrote an article entitled the *Quan Shi Lun* (*Exhortation*).

　　皇甫谧在搜求、阅读医书的过程中,感到现有针灸类医书对针灸学的承继、发展、传播十分不利。于是,他对比众多流传的针灸著作,删去重复部分,将相同内容予以归类,结合自己的实践,对精要内容详加论述,完成了《针灸甲乙经》,简称《甲乙经》。

　　《甲乙经》共12卷128篇,确定了654个穴位的正确部位,并对人体穴位按头、面、四肢、胸背等解剖部位进行了分类。详细记载了各个穴位的别名、所在部位、取穴方法、主治病症、针灸方法、针刺深度、留针时间、针灸禁忌等,形成完整、系统的经穴学,为学习医学者提供了读本和临床依据。

　　《甲乙经》在针灸学、临床医学和古医著的整理等方面都具有极高的学术价值,在中医学发展史上具有承前启后、继往开来的重要意义。

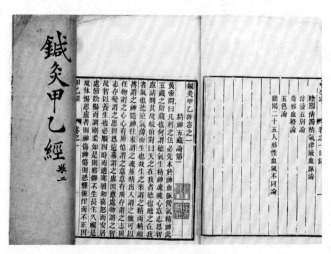

《针灸甲乙经》古籍
An Ancient Version of the *Zhenjiu Jiayi Jing*
(*A-B Classic of Acupuncture and Moxibustion*)

In the process of searching for and reading medical texts, Huangfu Mi realized that a lack of organization made it very unfavorable to the inheritance, development and dissemination of the knowledge about acupuncture and moxibustion. Therefore, he carefully reviewed existing acupuncture texts, eliminated redundant parts, categorized similar content from various texts, and expatiated some essential parts based on his own practice. Those efforts of his resulted in the completion of the *Zhenjiu Jiayi Jing* (*A-B Classic of Acupuncture and Moxibustion*), also called the *Jiayi Jing* for short.

The book consists of 12 volumes and 128 chapters, accurately identifying the locations of 654 acupuncture points and categorizing them according to various anatomical parts of the body, such as head, face, limbs, chest, and back. It also provides detailed information on the alternate names of the points, locations of each point, point selection, corresponding functions, needling techniques, depths of needling, retention times, and contraindications to the procedures. Providing a comprehensive and systematic description of acupuncture, this book serves as a fundamental textbook and clinical reference for medical learners.

The *Jiayi Jing* is of significant academic value in the fields of acupuncture, clinical medicine, and the compilation of ancient medical works. It plays a crucial role in the history of TCM, bridging the past, present and future in a line.

第二十章　敦煌医学名世界

敦煌,位于河西走廊的最西端,是丝绸之路的节点城市。在这里,除了有世界上现存规模最宏大、内容最丰富、保存最完好的石窟艺术宝库——莫高窟,还有与殷墟甲骨、居延汉简和明清档案并列为中国近代文化史上四大发现的"敦煌遗书"。"敦煌学"由此而来,而敦煌医学就是"敦煌学"中一颗璀璨的明珠。

据考证,敦煌医学资料的撰著年代最早可追溯到先秦和汉代,但绝大部分医书则是隋唐时代的著作。就医学内容而言,有医经诊法类、医术医方类、针灸药物类、养生类等。

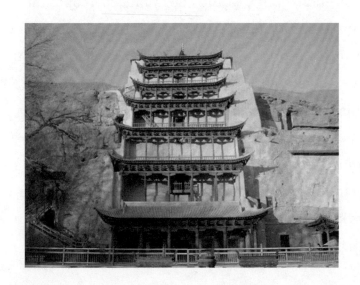

Chapter 20 World Famous Dunhuang Medicine

Dunhuang, located at the westernmost end of the Hexi Corridor, is a significant city along the Silk Road. In addition to its world-renowned Mogao Grottoes, which house the richest and best-preserved collection of cave art treasure with the largest scale, Dunhuang is also home to *Dunhuang Manuscripts*, considered one of the four major discoveries in modern Chinese cultural history alongside the oracle bones, *Juyan Han Jian*, and Archives of Ming and Qing dynasties. A discipline called "Dunhuang Studies" thus came into being, within which, Dunhuang medicine shines as a brilliant gem.

According to research, the earliest records of Dunhuang medical literature can be traced back to the pre-Qin and Han periods, but the majority of medical texts were written during the Sui and Tang dynasties. In terms of their medical content, they include categories such as medical classics and diagnostic methods, medical techniques and formulas, acupuncture, herbal medicine, and health preservation practices, etc.

例如,医经诊法类卷子包括《内经》《伤寒论》《脉经》的片段和托名张仲景的《五脏论》,以及《玄感脉经》《不知名脉法残片》《明堂五脏论》等十几种。内容涉及五脏、经脉、穴位的生理病理,有些是对《内经》等古籍的进一步补充和发挥,有些则是与传世古医籍不同的理论。医术医方类卷子有40多种,记载1000余首医方。内容涉及内、外、妇、儿、五官、皮肤等科。此外,还有大量美容长寿方,以及数十种外治法,如贴敷、熏洗、摩膏、溻渍等,充分体现了防治一体的学术思想。

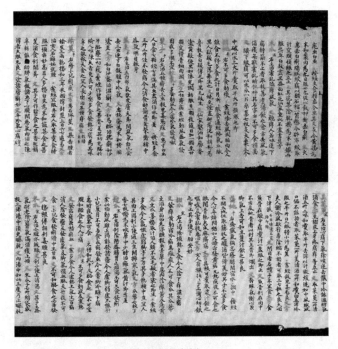

敦煌医学资料
Dunhuang Medical Literature

In the category of medical classics and diagnostic methods, there are a dozen volumes, including fragments from the *Huangdi Neijing*, *Shanghan Lun* (*Treatise on Exogenous Febrile Diseases*) and *Mai Jing* (*Pulse Classic*), as well as excerpts from the *Wuzang Lun* (*Reatise on the Five Zang-Organs*) attributed to Zhang Zhongjing, *Xuan Gan Mai Jing* (*Subtle Sensation and Pulse Diagnosis*), *Bu Zhiming Mai Fa Canpian* (*Fragmentation of Anonymous Sphygmology*), *Ming Tang Wuzang Lun* (*Reatise on the Five Zang-Organs of Ming and Tang Dynasties*), etc. The content covers the physiological and pathological aspects of five viscera, meridians, and points, some of which provide further elaboration on and supplement to ancient texts like the *Huangdi Neijing*, while others present theories different from those found in ancient medical books handed down from generation to generation. In the category of medical techniques and formulas, there are more than 40 volumes, containing over 1,000 medical formulas, whose content includes treatments for internal, external, gynecological, pediatric, ophthalmologic and otorhinolaryngologic diseases, and skin conditions, along with numerous formulas for beautification and longevity. Besides, there are dozens of external treatment methods offered such as plastering therapy, fuming-washing therapy, rubbing manipulation with ointment, wet compress and soaking, reflecting an integrated academic approach of combining prevention and treatment at the same time.

　　通过医学专家考察医方年代,认为其中除个别是见于前代医学方书的古方外,多是六朝、隋、唐代医家通过临床验证的有效验方。如《辅行诀脏腑用药法要》中载有五首救卒死中恶方,提到用硝石、雄黄散剂着舌下治疗中恶、急心痛、手足厥冷等方法,这比西方用硝酸甘油舌下含服治疗急性心肌梗死要早1000年。

　　此外,敦煌壁画也反映出古代劳动人民在生产与生活中同疾病做斗争的方式方法。如在敦煌壁画中就有治病救人、生病请医、讲究个人卫生、揩齿刷牙、运动和气功、洒扫庭院、拦护水井、剃头洗浴、建造厕所、煮沸食物等画面。

As for the origin of these medical prescriptions, it was confirmed by medical experts that a small number are ancient formulas that can be found in previous medical texts, and the majority are effective ones verified through clinical practice by medical practitioners during the Six dynasties, and the Sui and Tang dynasties. For instance, the *Fu Xing Jue Zangfu Yongyao Fa Yao* (*Auxiliary Notes on Medicines and Methods for Internal Organ Diseases*) lists five formulas for curing sudden fainting or sudden cardiac death, and one of them is to put saltpeter and *xionghuangsan* (realgar powder) under the patient's tongue to treat critical conditions, acute chest pain, and cold extremities. This method predates by 1,000 years the western practice of treating acute myocardial infarction with sublingual administration of nitroglycerin.

Furthermore, the Dunhuang murals also describe ancient laboring people fighting against diseases in their production and daily life. For example, in them one can find pictures of treating the sick and saving lives, seeking medical help, emphasizing personal hygiene, wiping teeth and brushing teeth, engaging in physical exercise and qigong, sweeping courtyards, guarding water wells, shaving heads and bathing, constructing toilets, and boiling food, etc.

敦煌医学大大丰富了隋唐前后的医学典籍，尤其丰富了魏晋南北朝的医学文献，反映了隋唐五代及前后医药学术成就，为古医籍的校勘和辑佚提供了重要资料，为医学史考证工作提供了有力的依据。

The records of Dunhuang medicine greatly contributed to the medical classics before and after the Sui and Tang dynasties, especially to the medical literature of the Wei, Jin, Southern and Northern dynasties, they reflect the achievements in medicine and pharmacology during the Sui, Tang, and Five dynasties, provide crucial information for the collation and restoration of ancient medical texts and offer strong evidence for the research and verification of the history of medicine in China.

第五单元　生活中的中医保健

　　中医药学发展了几千年，很多治疗技术随着文化交流扩散到世界各地，为世界各国的医学发展做了一定的贡献。中医养生，就是指通过各种方法颐养生命、增强体质、预防疾病，从而达到延年益寿的一种医事活动。中医养生重在整体性和系统性，目的是提前预防疾病，治未病。

　　进入青春期，青少年在体会很多成长的快乐的同时，也会有一些烦恼。在这个单元中，将介绍一些中医保健方面的知识，帮助大家保持良好的身心状态，以及饱满的精神状态投入到学习生活当中。

Unit V Health Preservation in Traditional Chinese Medicine

Traditional Chinese Medicine (TCM) has developed over thousands of years, and many treatments have spread worldwide with cultural exchanges, contributing to the medical advancements in many countries. Health preservation of TCM refers to a medical practice that helps people achieve longevity via maintaining a good health, enhancing physical fitness and preventing diseases through various methods. It focuses on integrity and systematicness, aiming at preventing diseases in advance and treating diseases before they manifest.

Approaching adolescence, teenagers will experience a lot of joy, and also some troubles in your life. In this unit, we will introduce some knowledge about TCM health preservation to help you maintain a good physical and mental state in your study and life.

同时,我们也结合青春期独有的生理心理特征,帮助大家掌握近视、长青春痘、肥胖等青少年常见的健康问题的防治方法。

希望大家通过学习,能够在以后的生活中运用好这些中医保健知识,这不但能够帮助自己缓解烦恼,也能帮助身边的亲人、朋友。现在,就让我们来领略中医保健在生活中的应用范例。

At the same time, considering the unique physiological and psychological characteristics of adolescence, we will offer some suitable ways to help you prevent and cope with some common health issues, such as myopia, acne and obesity.

We hope that you can apply such knowledge of TCM health preservation to your daily life after studying. This not only can help alleviate your own troubles, but also help your family and friends. Now, let us explore some examples of how to apply TCM health preservation in daily life.

第二十一章　饮食有节

宋代有位名医叫孙昉（fǎng），自号四休居士。有一天，黄庭坚问他为什么称"四休居士"？他笑笑回答说："吃的方面，不要过于讲究，只要吃得饱，粗茶淡饭就可以了；穿的方面，破了就补一补，只要能暖和，不觉得冷就可以了；家产呢，只要能过得去就行了；为人处世，既不贪图钱财，也不要嫉妒人家，能平平安安也就满足了。"黄庭坚非常称赞，并作诗纪念，因此为后人留下了"粗茶淡饭"的典故。

孙昉的养生理念，不仅启示我们生活要简朴，而且还告诉我们健康饮食的重要性。

《黄帝内经》中养生提倡的是一种健康的生活习惯，具体表现可以归为三个方面，即"饮食有节，起居有常，不妄作劳"。

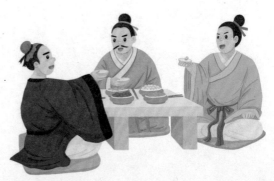

Chapter 21 Eating Moderately

In the Song dynasty, there was a famous doctor named Sun Fang, who took the title of Si Xiu Ju Shi (a scholar in seclusion who is moderate in four aspects). One day, Huang Tingjian asked him why he was called Si Xiu Ju Shi. He replied with a smile, "Don't pay too much attention to eating; as long as you have enough to eat, plain food is OK. In terms of clothing, mend it when it's torn, and it's adequate as long as it keeps you warm. In terms of family wealth, it's sufficient as long as you can get by. In dealings with others, do not be greedy for money, nor jealous of others, and be satisfied with peace. " Huang Tingjian thought highly of Sun's philosophy, and wrote a poem in his honor, leaving behind the story of "plain food" for later generations.

Sun's concept of health preservation not only inspires us to live simply, but also tells us the importance of a healthy diet.

The theory of health preservation in the *Huangdi Neijing* (*Huangdi's Classic of Medicine*) advocates a healthy lifestyle, to summarize, there are three main points, namely, "eating moderately, sleeping regularly, and avoiding excessive labor".

　　饮食有节，即饮食要有规律、有节制。《吕氏春秋》中说："食能以时，身必无灾。"《尚书》中也说"食哉唯时"。这两句话的大概意思，就是说按照一定时间有规律地进食，能使人体建立起条件反射，可以保证消化、吸收功能有规律地进行活动。我们传统的就餐时间是一日三餐，若能严格按时进食，不随便吃零食，养成良好的饮食习惯，则消化功能健旺，于身体健康大有益处。若不分时间，随意进食，零食不离口，就会使肠胃长时间工作，得不到休息，以致人体正常的消化规律被打破，久而久之可发生消化系统的疾病。

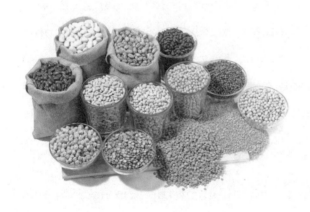

Firstly, we should eat regularly and in moderation. In the *Lüshi Chunqiu* (*Mr. Lü's Spring and Autumn Annals*), a compendium of the philosophies of the Hundred Schools of Thought, compiled around 239 BC under the patronage of the Qin dynasty chancellor Lü Buwei), it is said, "If you eat at the right time, no discomfort will occur to you." Similarly, it is mentioned in the *Shang Shu* (*Book of History*) that "One should eat at the right time." The general idea of these statements is that eating regularly at specific times can help establish conditioned reflexes in the body, ensuring that the digestion and absorption functions operate systematically. In traditional Chinese eating schedule, three meals a day are recommended. If you can eat strictly on time, avoid casual snacking, and develop good eating habits, your digestive function will be strong, which is of great benefit to your health. On the contrary, if you have your meals regardless of the time and eat snacks all the time, it will make your stomach overwork without any rest and disrupt your normal digestion, possibly leading to digestive disease over time.

第二十二章　起居有常

起居,即起卧作息与居住环境等生活的各个方面;有常,是指有一定的规律。起居有常主要指入睡和起床要有规律。每个人应根据季节的变化和自己的习惯,按时入睡,按时起床。

起居有常也包括有规律的生活,既合乎人体生理活动,也有利于维护中枢神经系统和植物神经系统的正常功能,使人体的新陈代谢正常,人的精神和身体就能循其道而长盛不衰。反之,如果一个人生活散漫,暴饮暴食,起居无常,对自己又恣意放纵,就会损伤身体健康。

Chapter 22 Rising & Resting Regularly

The second point is about having a regular daily life, which mainly refers to going to sleep and getting up regularly. Everyone should go to bed and get up on time according to seasonal changes and their habits.

Regular daily routine also includes a disciplined lifestyle, which not only aligns with human physiological activities but helps maintain the normal functions of the central nervous system and the autonomic nervous system, ensuring a normal metabolism in the body, when a person's mind and body follow this path, they will thrive and remain vigorous. Conversely, if one leads a disorderly life, eats and drinks too much, lacks regularity in daily routines, and indulges themselves, it will probably do harm to the body.

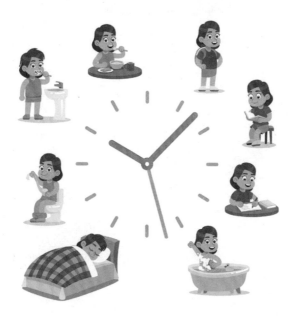

《黄帝内经》说："阳气尽则卧,阴气尽则寤(wù)。"说明睡眠与睡醒是阴阳交替的结果,阴气盛则入眠,阳气旺则醒来。子时是23时至1时,此时阴气最盛,阳气衰弱;午时是11时至13时,此时阳气最盛,阴气衰弱。

中医学认为,子时和午时都是阴阳交替之时,也是人体经气"合阴"与"合阳"的时候,睡好子午觉,有利于人体养阴、养阳。子时是一天中阴气最重的时候,这个时候休息,最能养阴,睡眠效果最好,而且睡眠质量最好,可以起到事半功倍的作用。这跟现代医学研究发现的人体需要在23点之前进入深睡眠状态的理论不谋而合。子时也是中医的经脉运行到肝、胆的时间,养肝的时间应该熟睡。如果因熬夜而错过了这个时间的睡眠,肝胆就得不到充分的休息,可表现为皮肤粗糙、黑斑、面色发黄等。

In the *Huangdi Neijing* (*Huangdi's Classic of Medicine*), it is stated, "When the yang qi is exhausted, then one falls asleep; when the yin qi is exhausted, then one is awake." This indicates that sleep and wakefulness are the results of the alternation of yin and yang. When the yin qi is abundant, one falls asleep, and when the yang qi is not plenty, one wakes up. At Zi Shi, the time from 23:00 to 1:00, the yin qi is at its peak and the yang qi the lowest point; while at Wu Shi, i.e. from 11:00 to 13:00, the yang qi is at its peak and the yin qi is the lowest point.

In the theory of Traditional Chinese Medicine (TCM), both Zi Shi and Wu Shi are times of transition between yin and yang, as well as moments when the meridian qi is harmonizing with yin and yang. A good sleep at midnight and a nap at noon are beneficial for nourishing both the yin and yang in the body. Zi Shi is the time when the yin qi is strongest during the day, and sleeping at this time can nourish the yin the most, leading to the best sleep quality and enhanced restorative effects. This aligns with the findings of modern medicine which suggests that human body should get into a state of deep sleep before 23:00. In TCM theory, Zi Shi is also the time when the meridians circulate into the liver and gallbladder, and a sound sleep can help nourish the liver. Staying up late and missing sleep during this time may lead to insufficient rest of the liver and gallbladder, and lead to symptoms like rough skin, dark spots, and a yellow complexion correspondingly.

午时"合阳"时间则要小寐,休息30分钟左右即可,最多不要超过1小时。即使不能够睡觉,也应"入静",使身体得以平衡过渡,提神醒脑、补充精力。我们来看个实例:居住在热带和地中海地区的人,比居住在北美和北欧的人患冠心病的概率要低,而前者恰恰就有午睡的习惯。科学家研究发现,24分钟的午睡,能够有效地改善驾驶员的注意力与表现。

睡子午觉还有几个注意事项:

1.天气再热也要在肚子上盖一点东西。

2.不要在有穿堂风的地方休息。

3.睡前最好不要吃太油腻的东西,因为这样会增加血液的黏稠度,加重心血管病变。

4.午休虽是打个盹,但也不可太随便,不要坐着或趴在桌子上睡,这会影响头部血液供应,导致醒后头昏、眼花、乏力。午休姿势应该是舒服地躺下,平卧或侧卧,最好的是头高脚低、向右侧卧。

Wu Shi is the time when the yang qi reaches the highest point of the day and the yin qi is about to rise gradually, and one is recommended to take a short nap during these two hours, preferably about 30 minute each and no more than 1 hour. Even if you can't fall asleep, you are advised to stay relatively motionless so that your body can adjust to the transition, refresh your mind and replenish your energy. For instance, people who live in the tropical and the Mediterranean regions have a lower risk of coronary heart disease compared to those living in North America and Northern Europe. The fact that the former have the habit of taking afternoon naps may produce this result. In addition, scientists have found that a 24-minute nap can effectively help a pilot stay focused during the flight.

Several do's and don'ts should be borne in mind when sleeping at Zi Shi and Wu Shi:

1. Cover your stomach with something even if the weather is hot.

2. Avoid resting in a place with a draft.

3. It is best not to eat greasy food before napping, as it may increase blood viscosity and aggravate cardiovascular diseases.

4. Do not sleep in a sitting posture or at a desk, as this can affect blood supply to the head, leading to dizziness, blurred vision and fatigue upon waking up. It is recommended to lie down comfortably during the nap, either flat or on the side, and the best posture is to lie on your right side, making your head slightly elevated and feet lowered.

　　人体的健康全靠有规律的"养"，只有遵循人体经脉气血运行的自然规律，"饮食有节，起居有常"，方能使身体达成和谐，进入健康佳境。

The health of the human body relies entirely on regular "nourishment". Only by following the natural laws of the circulation of qi and blood in the meridians of the human body, eating moderately and sleeping regularly, can you keep your body in a good condition and maintain an optimal state of health.

第二十三章　简易推拿

按摩又称推拿,是中国医学宝库中最具特色的一种医疗保健方法。它是施术者用双手或肢体的其他部位,在受术者的体表一定部位或穴位上施以各种手法操作,以达到防病治病、疏通经络等目的的一种物理疗法,以其简单易学、便于操作、疗效显著、费用低廉、无毒副反应等特点而备受人们的喜爱。

临床上按摩使用的手法种类很多,按其作用力的方向可分为下面五种。

推揉类:有推法、揉法、摩法、擦法、抹法等。

按拍类:有按法、掐法、拨法、振法、弹法、拍捶法、踩跷法等。

捏拿类:有捏法、拿法、搓法、提法等。

牵抖类:有抖法、引伸法等。

运动类:有屈伸法、摇法、扳法、背法等。

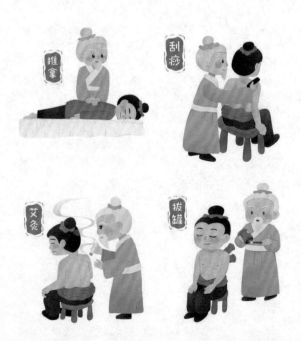

Chapter 23 Simple Massages

Massage, known as *tuina* in Chinese, is the most distinctive medical care method in the discipline of Traditional Chinese Medicine (TCM). It is a kind of physical therapy in which the practitioner uses hands or other parts of the body to perform various manipulations on certain body parts or acupoints of a patient. It can be used to prevent and treat diseases and unblock the meridian and collaterals. This physical therapy is welcomed because it is easy to learn and operate, remarkably effective, inexpensive and with no toxic side effects.

There are different massage techniques used in clinical practice, which can be divided into the following five categories according to the direction of force applied.

The first is pushing-kneading category, which mainly includes the pushing, kneading, rubbing, scrubbing and wiping manipulations, etc.

The second category is pressing and patting, including pressing, nipping, poking, vibrating, flicking, patting and pounding, treading and rolling, etc.

Pinching, grasping, twisting and lifting fall into the third category—the pinching-grasping manipulations.

The fourth, pulling-shaking category, includes the shaking manipulation and traction therapy, etc.

In the category of sports, there are stretching, rocking, pulling and back-packing manipulations.

各类推拿手法不同,所治疗的疾病也不相同,但都有舒筋活血、通经活络、缓解肌肉痉挛、解除肌肉酸痛、消除疲劳、扩张血管、加快血液循环等作用。

学会几招实用又简单的穴位推拿法非常有用,下面我们就来学一下吧。

按揉太阳穴。太阳穴在眉梢和外眼角中间,稍微往后一寸(约3.3厘米)凹陷部位。两手的食指指腹分别按住两侧太阳穴,顺时针和逆时针的方向依次按揉8次。能达到活络明目和祛风止痛效果,可辅助治疗头痛和眼疾。

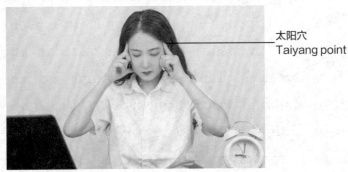

太阳穴
Taiyang point

掐内关穴。把手掌稍微仰起,手腕关节弯曲,手掌后第一横纹上两寸部位就是内关穴。用一手大拇指对此穴位按压,稍微用力,让局部感觉到酸胀为度,左右各按2分钟。可达到调和脾胃和宁心安神效果,同时也能活血通络和疏肝降逆。

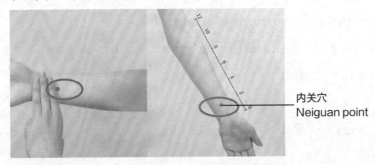

内关穴
Neiguan point

These massage techniques differ, and the diseases they treat are also different, but they all have the effects of relaxing sinews and activating blood circulation, unblocking the meridian and activating collaterals, relieving muscle spasms, alleviating muscle soreness, reducing fatigue, dilating blood vessels, and accelerating blood circulation, etc.

It is very useful to learn a few practical and simple acupoint massage techniques. Now let's do it.

First, press and knead the temples, which are located between the tip of the eyebrows and the outer corners of the eye, about 3 centimeters back in a sunken area. Use the pulms of your index fingers to press the temples on both sides, and knead them clockwise and counterclockwise, for 8 times each. This technique can help improve vision and activate collaterals, dispel wind and relieve pain, as well as assist in treating headaches and eye diseases.

Second, nip the neiguan point. Raise your palm slightly, bend the wrist joint, and you can find the neiguan point about 7 centimeters above the first transverse crease on the back of your palm. Use the thumb of one hand to press this point with a little force, to the extent that you can feel a slight soreness in this part, and press the point of each hand for 2 minutes. This manipulation can help harmonize the spleen and the stomach, calm the heart and tranquilize the mind, as well as promote blood circulation, free the collateral vessels, soothe the liver and alleviate nausea.

按涌泉穴。涌泉穴在足底掌心前面正中凹陷部位,一边洗脚,一边对涌泉穴按摩,每次各按摩5分钟,能促进肾脏健康,辅助治疗口腔溃疡和高血压。另外也能排毒养颜,促进脚部血液循环,温暖身体,防止呼吸道疾病。

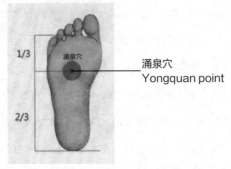

按摩耳轮。用两手的大拇指和食指分别捏住左右耳轮,从上往下不停搓摩,尽量让耳朵发热发胀最好。能达到活络通窍和聪耳明目效果,有利于全身健康。

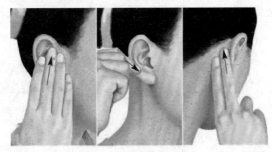

按摩耳轮
Massage the Helix

叩劳宫穴。首先把手握成拳头状,除了大拇指外,其他4个手指轻压掌心,无名指和中指两指间就是劳宫穴。把一手握成拳头状,用曲骨处叩击另一只手的劳宫穴,分别叩16次,能达到清热泻火和开窍醒神功效,还可去除心烦,辅助治疗心火旺盛所引起的口腔溃疡。

Then, press the yongquan point, which is in the middle of the sunken area in the front part of the sole. You can massage the points for 5 minutes each day while washing your feet. It can promote kidney health and assist in the treatment of oral ulcer and high blood pressure. In addition, it can also detoxify and beautify the skin, promote blood circulation in the feet, warm the body and prevent respiratory diseases.

Next, massage the helix. Pinch your left and right helices with your thumbs and forefingers of both hands, rub them from top to bottom, and try to make the ears hot and swollen. This can achieve the effects of promoting blood circulation, unblocking the orifices, and improving hearing and vision, which is beneficial to your overall health.

Fifth, tap the laogong point. When you clench your hand into a fist, use all your fingers except for the thumb to gently press the palm, you can find the laogong point right between the ring finger and the middle finger. Then, make a fist with one hand, and use the knuckles to tap the laogong point of the other hand, each hand for 16 times. It can help clear heat and purge fire, induce resuscitation and refresh mind, and remove vexation, as well as assist in the treatment of oral ulcer caused by exuberant heart fire.

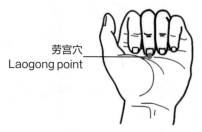

劳宫穴
Laogong point

按揉足三里穴。把膝盖弯曲成90度,从外膝盖眼向下量4横指,距离胫骨外一横指处部位就是足三里穴。大拇指指腹按摩此穴位,让局部有酸胀为主,每次按揉5分钟以上,能调理脾胃和气血,达到疏通经络和扶正培元效果,能辅助治疗胃肠道疾病,同时也能提高食欲,促进食物消化,改善心脏功能,帮助调节心律。

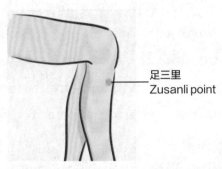

足三里
Zusanli point

掐睛明穴。端正坐好,轻轻闭上眼睛,目内眦稍上方凹陷处是睛明穴。用大拇指和中指掐在此穴位上,掐的时候一松一紧,点压2分钟,可达到疏风清热和通络明目效果,能辅助治疗神经性头痛、打嗝和眼疾。

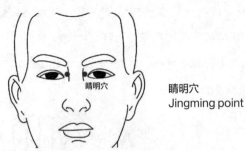

睛明穴

睛明穴
Jingming point

Next, press and knead the zusanli point. To locate this point, you have to bend the knee to 90 degrees and measure 4 horizontal fingers downward from the outer knee socket, and it's at the position one horizontal finger away from the outer edge of the shinbone. Use your thumb pulp to massage this point till you can feel the soreness, and make it last for more than 5 minutes each time. It can regulate the spleen and stomach, harmonize qi and blood, unblock the meridian and collateral vessels, reinforce the healthy qi and nurture the original qi. It can also assist in the treatment of gastrointestinal diseases and help improve appetite, promote food digestion, improve heart function and regulate heart rhythm.

Finally, nip the jingming point. Sit upright, close your eyes gently, and you can find jingming point above the inner canthus of your eyes. Nip the point with your thumb and middle finger, switching between forcefully and loosely, for 2 minutes. This has the effects of dispersing wind, clearing heat, freeing the collateral vessels and improving vision. In addition, it can assist in the treatments of neurogenic headaches, hiccups and eye diseases.

第二十四章　防控近视

近视是全球重大公共卫生问题,在中国呈低龄、高发、进展快的特征,已成为影响国民健康素质的重大问题。近视是指在调节放松状态下,来自5米以外的平行光线经眼球屈光系统后聚焦在视网膜之前的病理状态。

Chapter 24 Prevention and Control of Myopia

Myopia is a major global public health problem, characterized by a young age at onset, high incidence and rapid spread in China. It is now a major problem affecting the physical constitution of a large cohort of the population. Myopia refers to a pathological condition in which parallel light rays from 5 meters away focus in front of the retina after passing through the refractive system of the eyeball, under a relaxed state.

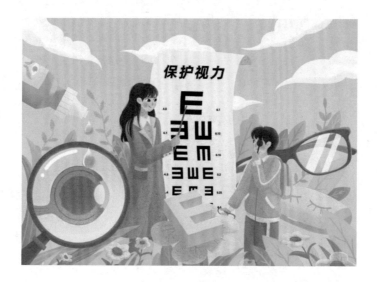

中医对近视早有研究。早在隋朝巢元方编撰的《诸病源候论》中,就已有"目不能远视"的记载,谓之"目不能远视,视物则茫茫漠漠也"。明代著名眼科医家傅仁宇在所著《审视瑶函》中,将此症命名为"能近怯远症",并有"久视伤睛成近觑"的记载。清代眼科名家黄庭镜在《目经大成》中明确了"近视"的概念。中医认为"五脏六腑之精气皆上注于目","目得血而能视",如果肝、脾、肾功能协调,精气充沛,自然目光敏锐。如果肝肾气血亏损,加上肠胃的运化功能失调,肾精不足,目失濡养,那么就会目视不明,从而造成近视。

There were studies on myopia in Traditional Chinese Medicine (TCM) back to the years. As early as in the Sui dynasty, in the *Zhu Bing Yuan Hou Lun* (*Treatise on Causes and Symptoms of Diseases*) by Chao Yuanfang, there was a record of shortsightedness, stating, "when the eyes cannot see distant objects clearly, everything appears vague and indistinct. " In the Ming dynasty, Fu Renyu, an eye specialist, depicted the symptom as "the disease of being able to see near but not far" in his book the *Shen Shi Yao Han* (*Examining Yao's Letter*, also called *A Complete Volume on Ophthalmology*), and wrote, "long-term eye strain hurts the eyes and leads to near-sightedness". In the Qing dynasty, Huang Tingjing, a famous ophthalmologist, defined the concept of "short-sightedness" in his *Mu Jing Da Cheng* (*A Book on Eye Disorders & Diseases*). It is believed in TCM that "the essence and energy of the five viscera and six bowels are concentrated in the eyes", and "the eyes can see when nourished by blood". When the functions of the liver, spleen, and kidneys are coordinated, and the essence and energy abundant, a person can have a sharp vision accordingly. In contrary, if the liver and kidney are deficient in qi and blood, and there exists a dysfunction in the digestive system and insufficiency in kidney essence, the eyes would lose its clear vision because of the lack of nourishment, which may result in myopia.

《黄帝内经》说"目不劳，心不惑，才能游行天地之间，视听八达之外"，所以保护眼睛最重要的是要避免"久视伤血"。近距离用眼姿势是影响近视眼发生率的另一个因素，近距离用眼时，身体应保持静止状态，坐姿端正，书本放在距眼睛30厘米左右的地方。乘车、躺在床上、或伏案歪头阅读等不良习惯都会增加眼的调节负担，增加眼外肌对眼球的压力，尤其是中小学生的眼球正处于发育阶段，长时间的不良用眼姿势容易引起眼球的发育异常，导致近视眼的形成。应端正看书写字的姿势，写字时，光线最好从左前方照到书本，避免写字时光线被右手挡住。看电视时注意高度应与视线相平；眼与电视的距离大于荧光屏对角线长的5～6倍，且室内应有一定的背景光。

It is said in the *Huangdi Neijing* (*Huangdi's Classic of Medicine*) that "Only when the eyes are not tired and the mind not confused, one can wander around and be widely informed". The most important thing to protect one's eyes is to avoid a "long-term eye strain", because it may cause blood deficiency. Another factor that may cause myopia is short-distanced use of eyes. When using the eyes at a short distance, you should keep your body still, sit upright, and place the book about 30 centimeters away from your eyes. Do not read while riding or when you lie on the bed, and do not read with a tilted head, because bad reading habits will increase the burden of eye adjustment and increase the pressure of extraocular muscles on the eyeball. Especially for you teenagers, whose eyeballs are still in a developmental stage, a long-term bad posture is easy to cause an abnormal development of the eyeball, leading to shortsightedness. Thus, it is important for you to maintain a proper posture when reading or writing. When writing, you'd better ensure that the light comes from the upper left side, so as to avoid the light being blocked by your right hand. When watching TV, make sure the set is at your sight level, the distance between the eyes and the TV is 5-6 times longer than the diagonal length of the fluorescent screen, and there should be a certain amount of background light in the room.

　　对于青少年来说,看电脑的时间过长也会造成眼睛调节痉挛,从而造成近视。看书或使用电脑2小时后,一定要休息10~15分钟,此时可远眺窗外景观,或转动眼球、做眼保健操等,只要不集中在近距离用眼,都有休息效果。每天早晨起来,要在空气新鲜中闭目养神,眼球从右到左,再从左到右各转5次,然后依次注视左、右、右上角、左上角、右下角、左下角,反复5次,然后睁开眼睛,极目远眺。多看看远处的风景,对眼睛是有好处的。手机、电脑、电视,以及数码产品的LED屏幕有高能蓝光,蓝光是一种穿透力很强的可见光,过长时间照射对人眼有害,正在发育中的青少年要尽量缩短看屏幕的时间。

　　为了让中医适宜技术防控儿童青少年近视,中华中医药学会特制定了《中医适宜技术耳穴压丸防控儿童青少年近视操作指南》,孩子们可以在医生指导下学习操作。

For teenagers, spending too much time looking at a computer screen can cause eye accommodation spasms, leading to myopia. After reading or using a computer for 2 hours, it is essential to take a 10-15 minutes break. During this time, look into the distance at the scenery outside, move your eyes around, or do eye exercises. As long as you are not focusing on close-range vision, any activity can have a restorative effect. Every morning, try to do the following exercises: first, have your eyes closed and refresh your mind. Then, move your eyes from right to left and then left to right five times each. Next, look at the left, right, upper right corner, upper left corner, lower right corner, and lower left corner sequentially, with your eyes still closed, and repeat that five times. Finally, open your eyes and look into the distance. Looking at the scenery in the distance is good for the eyes. While the high-energy blue light found in LED screens of mobile phones, computers, televisions and digital products, which is a kind of visible light with a strong penetrating power, is harmful to human eyes with prolonged exposure, teenagers in the developmental stage should try to shorten the time of looking at the screen.

In order to apply suitable techniques in TCM to the prevention and control of myopia in children and adolescents, the China Association of Chinese Medicine has formulated *The Operational Guidelines for the Prevention and Control of Myopia in Children and Adolescents through Appropriate Techniques of Traditional Chinese Medicine—Auricular Point Plaster Therapy.* Teenagers can learn the manipulating methods under the guidance of doctors.

耳穴压丸防控儿童青少年近视操作规范：

1.材料：王不留行。

2.取穴：（单耳操作）

主穴：肝、脾、心、肾穴。

配穴：眼、目1、目2、神门穴，以上穴位任选

1～2穴。

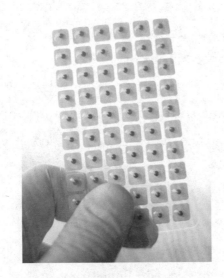

王不留行耳穴贴

Cowherb Seed Ear Acupuncture Sticker

Operation specifications for prevention and control of myopia in children and adolescents by the auricular point plaster therapy:

1. Material: *wangbuliuxing* (cowherb seed).

2. acupoint selection: (monaural operation)

Main points: liver, spleen, heart and kidney.

Matching points: eye1, eye 2, shenmen point, select one or two points at a time.

Schematic diagram:

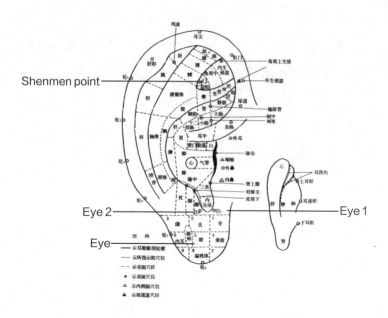

耳穴国际标准化方案穴区分布示意图

The Auricular Points Chart in the *Auricular Acupuncture Point* (in 2011)

第二十五章　传统保健

中医药学一直以来重视个体的养生和预防保健，提倡运用多种传统保健功法来调理身心，从而达到强身健体、延年益寿的目的。其中，最古老、最有影响的保健功法有五禽戏、太极拳、马王堆导引术、八段锦、易筋经等。

Chapter 25 Traditional Health Care

Traditional Chinese Medicine (TCM) has always attached great importance to individual health preservation, disease prevention and health care. Many traditional health exercises are advocated to regulate the body and mind, so as to strengthen the physical health and prolong life. Among them, the oldest and most influential exercises are the wuqinxi (a set of physical exercises imitating the movements of the five animals), tai chi (shadowboxing), the Mawangdui daoyinshu (physical and breathing exercises recorded on silk unearthed from the Mawangdui Han Tomb), the baduanjin (eight-sectioned exercise), the yijinjing (rejuvenating exercise) and so on.

　　五禽戏相传是华佗创制的一种外动内静、动中求静的功法，习练时应做到外动内静，动中求静，刚柔并举；练内练外，内外兼备；有动有静，动静相兼。可单练一禽之戏，也可选练一两个动作。五禽戏有五种类型的动作，各类典型动作有：虎寻食、鹿长跑、熊撼运、猿摘果、鹤飞翔等。练时要求模仿得逼真，不仅形似，而且神似，如虎的威猛扑动，鹿的伸颈回首，猿的机灵敏捷，熊的深厚沉稳，鸟的展翅翘立。

　　据史书记载，华佗的徒弟吴普坚持练习五禽戏，90多岁了，还耳聪目明，牙齿坚固不掉。

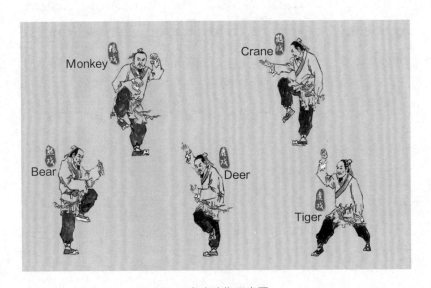

五禽戏动作示意图
Schematic Diagram of the Wuqinxi
(In the above pictures, people are doing the movements that imtate the motion of the bear, monkey, deer, crane and tiger.)

Legend has it that the wuqinxi was created by Hua Tuo. It is an exercise combining physical movement with inner peace, seeking peace in movement. When practicing, one should keep inner peace in every move, strengthen the body with soft actions and integrate movement with stillness. You can choose one section to practice, or just one or two movements. There are five sections in the wuqinxi, corresponding to five animals, and the typical movements in each section include tiger looking for food, deer running, bear shaking, ape picking fruit and crane flying, etc. When practicing, you should imitate the animal in a lifelike way, not only in shape, but also in spirit, such as the fierce attack of the tiger, the agility and vigilance of the deer, the quick-wittedness of the ape, the calmness and composure the bear and the vitality and lightness of the bird.

According to historical records, Wu Pu, a disciple of Hua Tuo, who had persisted in practicing the wuqinqi for years, still had sharp hearing, clear eyesight, and strong teeth in his 90s.

　　太极拳是以中国传统儒、道哲学中的太极、阴阳辨证理念为核心思想，集颐养性情、强身健体、技击对抗等多种功能于一体，结合易学的阴阳五行之变化，中医经络学，古代的导引术和吐纳术形成的一种内外兼修、柔和、缓慢、轻灵、刚柔相济的中国传统拳术。

　　1949年之后，太极拳被国家体委（现为国家体育总局）统一改编，作为强身健体的体操运动，增加了表演、体育比赛用途。后来分为比武用的太极拳、体操运动用的太极操和太极推手。

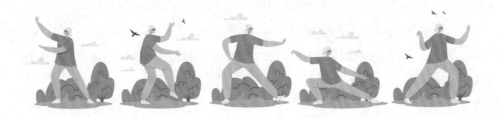

　　传统太极拳门派众多，常见的太极拳流派有陈式、杨式、武式、吴式、孙式、和式等，各派既有传承关系，相互借鉴，也各有自己的特点，呈百花齐放之态。由于太极拳是近代形成的拳种，流派众多，群众基础广泛，因此是中国武术拳种中非常具有生命力的一支。2020年，联合国教科文组织将"太极拳"项目列入人类非物质文化遗产代表作名录。

Tai chi is a kind of traditional Chinese boxing based on the core idea of tai chi (meaning supreme ultimate) and yin and yang dialectics in the traditional Confucian and Taoist philosophy. It integrates many functions such as selfcultivating, body building, fighting and confronting. It combines the changes of yin and yang, and the Five Elements in yiology (philosophy in *Book of Changes*), science of channels and collaterals in TCM and physical and breathing exercises in ancient China to form a kind of traditional Chinese boxing with a cultivation of both the internal and external, characterized by slowness, lightness and a coupling of hardness with softness.

After 1949, tai chi was unified and adapted by the National Sports Commission (now called General Administration of Sport of China) as a gymnastics exercise for improving health and fitness, with added application in performance and sports competitions. It was later divided into martial art tai chi, tai chi gymnastics, and tai chi pushing hands for different purposes.

There are many traditional tai chi schools, with common styles including Chen, Yang, Wǔ, Wú, Sun, and He, etc. Different schools have been inheriting and learning from others, while each has its own characteristics, presenting a diverse and flourishing state. As tai chi is a modern form with numerous schools and a wide popular base, it is a vital branch in Chinese martial arts. In 2020, UNESCO included the "tai chi" project in the Representative List of the Intangible Cultural Heritage of Humanity.

　　1974年，在长沙马王堆汉墓中出土了一幅彩色帛图，经过专家们的拼合糊裱，发现是一幅记载古人锻炼身体的养生图，即现在的《马王堆导引图》，它记录的马王堆导引术是中国最古老的健身项目。

　　《马王堆导引图》是中国现存最早的一幅健身图谱，距今已有几千年历史。它的发现填补了中国从春秋战国时期到西汉时期导引术的一段空白。它结合了中国古老的中医学、养生学以及自然美学，其中许多动作模拟动物形态，如"龙登""鹤舞"，动作优美，衔接流畅，循经导引，行意相随。练习后能调和气息，平衡阴阳，顺畅血液循环。是一套古朴优美、内外兼修，集修身、养性、娱乐、观赏于一体的健身之法。

　　国家体育总局依据《马王堆导引图》，从中选取17个动作，组编成了"马王堆导引术"，适合不同人群练习，具有祛病强身、延年益寿的功效。

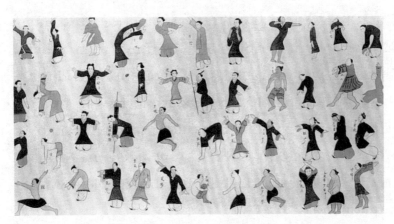

马王堆汉墓出土导引图复原图

A Restored Picture of the *Mawangdui Daoyin Diagram*

In 1974, a colored silk painting was unearthed from the Mawangdui Han Tomb in Changsha. It was pieced and pasted together by experts, and turned out to be a health-maintaining diagram, known as the *Mawangdui Daoyin Diagram*, showing how ancient people did physical exercises. The Mawangdui daoyinshu, the fitness exercise shown in the diagram, is believed to be the oldest in China.

The *Mawangdui Daoyin Diagram* is the earliest fitness diagram found in China, with a history of thousands of years. Its discovery filled in the blank of daoyinshu (conduction exercise) in China from the Spring and Autumn period to the Western Han dynasty. It combines ancient Chinese medicine, health preservation practices, and natural aesthetics, with many movements mimicking animal behaviors, such as "dragon ascending" and "crane dancing", being graceful in movements and smooth in a cohesion. Practicing these exercises can harmonize breathing, balance yin and yang, and promote smooth circulation of blood. It is a set of ancient and elegant exercises that integrate internal and external cultivation, encompassing physical fitness, mental cultivation, entertainment, and aesthetic appreciation.

The State Sport General Administration selected 17 movements from the *Mawangdui Daoyin Diagram*, and compiled them into the Mawangdui daoyinshu, making it suitable for different people to practice to eliminate diseases, strengthen the body and prolong life.

八段锦功法是一套独立而完整的健身功法，起源于北宋时期，已有900多年的历史了。在中国古老的引导术中，八段锦是流传最广、对导引术发展影响最大的一种。

八段锦一般有八节，锦是由"金""帛"组成，以表示其精美华贵。现代的八段锦在内容与名称上均有所改变。此功法分为八段，每段一个动作，练习无需器械，不受场地局限，简单易学，节省时间，作用极其显著，适合于男女老少。

2020年，国家中医药管理局印发《新型冠状病毒肺炎恢复期中医康复指导建议（试行）》，其中提到：新冠肺炎轻型、普通型、重型或危重型患者出院后，可以根据自身恢复情况选择适当的传统功法，自我干预，促进恢复。而其中首选的传统功法便是八段锦。

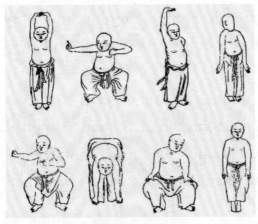

八段锦动作示意图
Schematic Diagram of Baduanjin

The baduanjin (meaning "eight silk brocade" in Chinese) is an independent and complete set of fitness exercises and originated in the Northern Song dynasty more than 900 years ago. Of the Chinese ways of exercises, the baduanjin is the most widely spread and most highly influential one.

In general, the baduanjin consists of eight parts (ba duan in Chinese meaning "eight parts or pieces") of exercises. The Chinese character "锦" (*jin*) is composed of "金" (gold) and "帛" (silk), which expresses a feeling of exquisite luxury. The modern version of the baduanjin has changed in both the content and name. It is divided into eight sections, with each section consisting of a single movement. It can be practiced without the need of any equipment or limitation of the site, and it is time-saving, simple and easy to learn, suitable for men, women, old and young.

In 2020, the National Administration of TCM issued the *Guidelines for Recovery by Using TCM Methods in the Convalescent Period of COVID-19 (Trial Version)*, suggesting that discharged patients who had mild, ordinary, severe or critical COVID-19 can choose appropriate traditional exercises and do self-intervention to promote recovery. Of the traditional exercises, the baduanjin is the best choice.

213